ABC of
Domestic and Sexual Violence

T0176621

ABC series

An outstanding collection of resources for everyone in primary care

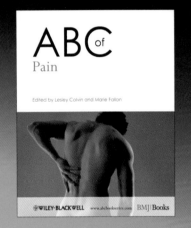

ABC of Pain

Edited by Lesley Colvin and Marie Fallon

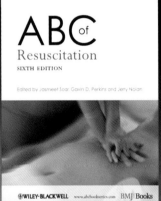

ABC of Resuscitation

SIXTH EDITION

Edited by Jasmeet Soar, Gavin D. Perkins and Jerry Nolan

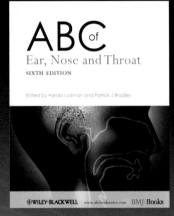

ABC of Ear, Nose and Throat

SIXTH EDITION

Edited by Harold Ludman and Patrick J Bradley

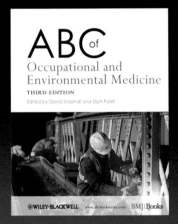

ABC of Occupational and Environmental Medicine

THIRD EDITION

Edited by David Snashall and Dipti Patel

The *ABC* series contains a wealth of indispensable resources for GPs, GP registrars, junior doctors, doctors in training and all those in primary care

▶ **Highly illustrated, informative and a practical source of knowledge**

▶ **An easy-to-use resource, covering the symptoms, investigations, treatment and management of conditions presenting in day-to-day practice and patient support**

▶ **Full colour photographs and illustrations aid diagnosis and patient understanding of a condition**

For more information on all books in the *ABC* series, including links to further information, references and links to the latest official guidelines, please visit:

www.abcbookseries.com

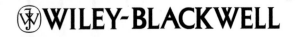

WILEY-BLACKWELL

BMJ|Books

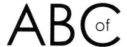

ABC of
Domestic and Sexual Violence

EDITED BY

Susan Bewley

Women's Health Academic Centre
King's College London
UK

Jan Welch

Caldecot Centre
King's College Hospital NHS Foundation Trust
UK

and

South Thames Foundation School
UK

WILEY Blackwell

BMJ Books

This edition first published 2014 © 2014 by John Wiley & Sons, Ltd.

BMJ Books is an imprint of BMJ Publishing Group Limited, used under licence by John Wiley & Sons.

Registered office: John Wiley & Sons, Ltd, The Atrium, Southern Gate, Chichester, West Sussex, PO19 8SQ, UK

Editorial offices: 9600 Garsington Road, Oxford, OX4 2DQ, UK

The Atrium, Southern Gate, Chichester, West Sussex, PO19 8SQ, UK

111 River Street, Hoboken, NJ 07030-5774, USA

For details of our global editorial offices, for customer services and for information about how to apply for permission to reuse the copyright material in this book please see our website at www.wiley.com/wiley-blackwell

Library of Congress Cataloging-in-Publication Data

ABC of domestic and sexual violence / edited by Susan Bewley, Jan Welch.
    p. ; cm.
  Includes bibliographical references and index.
   ISBN 978-1-118-48218-6 (paperback)
  I. Bewley, Susan, editor of compilation. II. Welch, Jan editor of compilation.
  [DNLM: 1. Domestic Violence. 2. Sex Offenses. 3. Battered Women. 4. Crime Victims. WA 308]
  RC569.5.F3
  616.85'822–dc23
                                                      2013044785

A catalogue record for this book is available from the British Library.

Wiley also publishes its books in a variety of electronic formats. Some content that appears in print may not be available in electronic books.

Cover image: Photograph by Jade Turnbull, Copyright © 2014, Jade Photography
Cover Design by Andy Meaden.

Set in 9.25/12pt Minion by Laserwords Private Ltd, Chennai, India
Printed and bound in Malaysia by Vivar Printing Sdn Bhd

1 2014

Contents

Contributors

Gwen Adshead
Forensic Psychiatry
Southern Health Foundation Trust
UK

Rasha Al Dabaan
Department of Pediatric Dentistry and Orthodontics
King Saud University, College of Dentistry
Saudi Arabia

Loraine J. Bacchus
Department of Global Health and Development
Gender Violence and Health Centre
London School of Hygiene & Tropical Medicine
UK

Jackie Barron
Women's Aid Federation of England
UK

Susan Bewley
Women's Health Academic Centre
King's College London
UK

Nicole Biros
Victim Witness Advocacy
Boost Child Abuse Prevention and Intervention
Canada

Emmeline Brew-Graves
General Practice
Southway Surgery
UK

Bernadette Butler
The Haven Camberwell Sexual Assault Referral Centre
King's College Hospital NHS Foundation Trust
UK

Wendy Cottee
Crown Prosecution Service
UK

Sarah M. Creighton
Department of Women's Health
University College London Hospital
UK

Maureen Dalton
SARC Commissioning South West
UK

Fiona Duxbury
General Practice
Oxford
UK

Gene Feder
Centre for Academic Primary Care
School of Social and Community Medicine
University of Bristol
UK

Colin Fitzgerald
Respect
UK

Andrea Goddard
Department of Paediatrics
Imperial College London
UK

Louise M. Howard
Institute of Psychiatry
King's College London
UK

Emma Howarth
Centre for Academic Primary Care
School of Social and Community Medicine
University of Bristol
UK

Medina Johnson
Next Link Domestic Abuse Services
UK

Michael King
Mental Health Sciences Unit
University College London Medical School
UK

Marai Larasi
Imkaan
UK

Hannah Loftus
Genitourinary Medicine
Sheffield Teaching Hospitals NHS Foundation Trust
UK

Finbarr C. Martin
Department of Geriatrics
Guys and St Thomas' NHS Trust
UK

Ali Mears
Genitourinary Medicine and HIV
Imperial College Healthcare NHS Trust
UK

Tim Newton
Dental Institute
King's College London
UK

Karen Rogstad
Genitourinary Medicine
Sheffield Teaching Hospitals NHS Foundation Trust
UK

Alex Sohal
Centre for Primary Care and Public Health
Queen Mary University of London
UK

Lindsey Stevens
Department of Emergency Medicine
Epsom and St Helier University NHS Trust
UK

Fiona Subotsky
Royal College of Psychiatrists
UK

Jo Todd
Respect
UK

Eleanor Turner Moss
Barts and The London School of Medicine and Dentistry
Queen Mary University of London
UK

Jan Welch
Caldecot Centre
King's College Hospital NHS Foundation Trust
UK and
South Thames Foundation School
UK

Catherine White
Sexual Assault Referral Centre
St Mary's Manchester
UK

Foreword

Sir George Alberti

King's College Hospital NHS Foundation Trust, UK

Domestic and sexual violence have almost certainly been with us ever since human history began. For centuries they have been largely ignored and even now all we see is the tip of the iceberg. Fortunately more attention is now focused on them as major societal problems. Nonetheless there is still widespread ignorance, particularly in the health professions, as to the nature and scale of the problem. I recently chaired a Department of Health Taskforce on Violence Against Women and Children and was appalled by the numbers of people affected – not just by serious sexual crimes but also by all forms of domestic violence. I was particularly impressed by the numbers of unrecognised cases in general practice, emergency departments and hospital outpatient services even when obvious triggers were present – with some notable exceptions.

I was also disappointed by the lack of attention given to sexual and domestic violence in medical school curricula and postgraduate training programmes. There should be much more focus on multidisciplinary working with close contact between different agencies. Often mechanisms are in place but are underused.

The Taskforce brought some attention to the issues involved but did not solve the many problems. The present volume goes some way to rectifying this. It is a superb vade mecum which should be required reading at an early stage for all health professionals but particularly those working in general practice and long-term conditions. It should also be freely used in training health care professionals. I cannot commend it to you strongly enough!

Introduction

Susan Bewley[1] and Jan Welch[2,3]

[1]Women's Health Academic Centre, King's College London, UK
[2]Caldecot Centre, King's College Hospital NHS Foundation Trust, UK
[3]South Thames Foundation School, UK

Purpose

Why do health care professionals need to know about domestic and sexual violence? Surely these are either private issues or someone else's business (e.g. the police)? In recent years it has increasingly been recognised that this is not the case. 'Privacy' has allowed serious crime to go undetected and perpetrators to act with impunity. Health care professionals look after patients whose lives are blighted by violence and abuse, whose health is impacted – and who can be helped if the professionals understand how.

Even though domestic and sexual violence affect far more people than do conditions such as diabetes and inflammatory bowel disease, they have featured much less on medical school and postgraduate curricula, and are sometimes entirely absent. Many doctors are not aware of how common these problems are, how to identify them or what to do next. This book aims to provide practical support to learners early in their careers.

Historical perspective

Allusions to domestic and sexual violence occur in some of the earliest written works and feature in ancient stories, such as the rape of Antiope by the Greek king of the gods and sexual predator Zeus. While rape was recognised as a crime in ancient Rome, 'wife beating' for correctional purposes was criminalised only much more recently and remains the norm in some cultures today. Rape is an expression of power. It has long been both a weapon of war and a means of oppressing the vanquished – men as well as women. Following the capture of Berlin by the Red Army in 1945, an estimated 2 million German women and girls were raped by Soviet troops. More recently, in the Rwandan genocide of 1994, many thousands of Tutsi women were subjected to rape, many acquiring HIV as a result. Some were also sexually mutilated in order to destroy their future reproductive capabilities.

Women's position in society has changed over the centuries. In most countries, women are no longer considered to be legal minors: the possessions initially of their fathers and then of their husbands. Attitudes to violence against women have changed in parallel and legislation has followed; for example, during the last 30 years marital rape has been criminalised in most Western countries.

Modern relevance

Sadly, abuse and rape remain common in modern societies, whether resource-poor or heavily industrialised. Much is covert, as victims experience fear and shame, which often inhibit disclosure. Many victims wait until the right moment to disclose – perhaps to a practitioner they trust. The health impacts can be immediate or can only become evident much later. In the UK each week two women are killed by their partners, but this is just the tip of the iceberg: many more seek help for nonspecific physical symptoms or mental health problems related to previous abuse.

While anyone can be assaulted or abused, the presence of co-vulnerabilities increases the likelihood. Perpetrators are adept at identifying those with vulnerabilities, whether long-term (e.g. learning or other disability), situational (e.g. being in a conflict zone) or transient (e.g. when someone is under the influence of alcohol or drugs).

Language

Language is dynamic and nomenclature can be problematic, as words inevitably carry connotations (or 'baggage') with them. For example, some writers prefer the term 'abuse' to 'violence' as it is more inclusive; it may make it clearer that the damage is not merely physical, but mental, lasting longer than the processes of physical healing and going deeper than the outward, superficial scars.

The term 'survivor' is generally preferred to 'victim' when discussing people who have been subjected to domestic violence, as it recognises the individual strength necessary to carry on in difficult circumstances and often to protect others, such as children. When encountering people who have suffered extreme human rights abuses or torture at the hands of others, however, this could seem trite.

'Empowerment' might be trivialised by cosmetic product advertising slogans ('because you're worth it'), but is a real process for the most disadvantaged, abused and voiceless members of society. Other terms, including 'patient', 'complainant' and 'client', vary in their suitability and acceptability. Although there are gender differences in the perpetration and experience of violence, abuse has no limits for people of any age, sex, race, sexuality, class, creed or political persuasion.

The National Health Service has a 'universalist' perspective; that is, it is available to all on the basis of need. We have tried to maintain this stance throughout, although most case studies refer to women and children. The chapter authors come from a wide variety of backgrounds: professional and voluntary sector; medical, legal, academic and lay. They bring different values and 'cultures' with them, reflecting the fact that a multi-agency response is required for these persistent societal wrongs. Thus, although terminology varies throughout the book, we have tried to ensure that the words used are appropriate for the context, while recognising that others may disagree.

We hope that the variety of examples of questions and responses given in the chapters will act as templates while you develop your own strategies and practice styles. Reflective practitioners pay careful attention to the exact words patients use, as well as to gaps, silences and alignments with nonverbal cues. They also choose their words carefully, while modulating their tone and body language, in order to build rapport, diminish fear, overcome stigma and prejudice and demonstrate trustworthiness. Lessons learned from this book can be applied to many other settings.

The role of doctors

It is important for future good doctors to recognise their role, which is to *recognise*, *empathise* and *witness* and to *refer* to appropriate multi-agency services. Violence does not fit the traditional 'medical model' of diagnosis, prognosis and plan, and should not be 'medicalised' as something that can be 'fixed' by doctors using conventional treatments. However, it may coexist with other conventional comorbidities, may explain patient presentations and behaviours and may interfere with the ability of patients to trust or comply with their doctor's advice.

Uncovering our patients' narrative, or story, may make sense of otherwise unresolvable medical presentations (and explain the old maxim that 'there is no such thing as a difficult patient, only a patient with difficult problems'). Even when there are time constraints, or when patients are unwilling to talk or disclose, an acknowledgment can help a patient feel known and understood. Kindness costs nothing; compassion takes no time. They may make all the difference to a vulnerable person feeling empowered to speak now or at a later date. Whether abuse, violence, mental illness, substance misuse or another 'life problem' lurks in your patient's or their family's background, failure to respond sensitively may lead to misattribution or dismissal of symptoms, misdiagnosis of disease, repeated inappropriate investigation and at worst, retraumatisation or even abuse by professionals.

Boundaries and difficult issues

Both patients' and doctors' interests are protected by the vital professional promises of confidentiality and boundaries of consent. It is within these formal, legally and professionally binding constraints of the doctor–patient relationship that value, skills and even creativity lie. Only very occasionally can they be broken, and this must only be done with transparency and senior and expert support.

Some readers will inevitably have experienced violence themselves, first-hand or in their friends and families, or will experience it in the future, either on the giving or the receiving end. Doctors may be fearful of involvement with the topic or may have personal concerns for their own safety. Alternatively, they may be fearful of raising concerns about patients or team dynamics if they fear reprisals or are being bullied at work. Doctors may find they feel powerful negative emotions towards patients, including hostility, anger or frustration, or even unanticipated or inappropriate feelings of intimacy or attraction. The art of professionalism is to recognise and control these feelings, to put them to one side and not to act on them. But we are not automatons. We need quiet time and 'headspace' to recover and reflect both 'on practice' and 'within practice'. '*What do such feelings say about the patient and about me, the practitioner?*' '*What do the team behaviours, dynamics and "jokes" say about us and our ability to empathise?*' '*Where can I find reliable sources of support, learning, guidance and wisdom?*'

Lifelong learning

As doctors who had virtually no knowledge of or training in domestic and sexual violence as students, we learnt the hard way – from our patients and from our mistakes, by trial and error and by carving out services and research from scratch. Looking back over our combined 6 decades of medical practice, we dreamt of a book that we wished had existed when we started out. Although few readers will end up majoring in responses to violence (as we have), everyone will encounter it – whether explicit or hidden – in the clinics and wards, and everyone can make a positive health contribution. Our authors have distilled their accumulated wisdom in the hope of accelerating your learning and making you better practitioners. We hope that the lessons in this book will stand you in good stead and that you find fulfilling careers wherever you end up. Keeping the care of your patient as your first concern and safety at the forefront of your mind will also act as a reliable guide.

CHAPTER 1

The Epidemiology of Gender-Based Violence

Gene Feder and Emma Howarth

Centre for Academic Primary Care, School of Social and Community Medicine, University of Bristol, UK

OVERVIEW

- The most consistent risk factor for domestic and sexual violence is being a woman; most severe domestic violence and most sexual violence is perpetrated by men
- Hence, sexual and domestic violence are gender-based, although men can also be victims of interpersonal violence
- The term 'gender-based violence' highlights the roots of violence against women in gender inequality
- Gender-based violence is both a breach of human rights and a major challenge to public health and clinical practice

---

What are domestic violence and sexual violence and why are they gender-based?

This chapter outlines the epidemiology of gender-based violence in the UK and internationally in terms of prevalence, community vulnerability and health impact. It concludes with reflections on why it remains so hidden from doctors and other clinicians and the need for robust research on effective health care responses.

In the UK, domestic violence is defined as any incident or pattern of incidents of controlling, coercive or threatening behaviour, violence or abuse between people aged 16 or over who are or have been intimate partners or family members, regardless of gender or sexuality.

This can encompass, but is not limited to, the following types of abuse:

- Psychological.
- Physical.
- Sexual.
- Financial.
- Emotional.

Sexual violence is a major component of domestic violence, often co-occurring with other forms of abuse, and includes sexual abuse from carers, strangers, acquaintances or friends. It is defined as any sexual act, attempt to obtain a sexual act, unwanted sexual comment or advance, attempt to traffic, or other act directed against a person's sexuality using coercion, by any person regardless of their relationship to the victim, in any setting.

Gender-based violence is not confined to domestic and sexual violence. It includes:

- Female genital mutilation (see Chapter 17).
- Femicide, including (so-called) honour- and dowry-related killings (see Box 3.2).
- Human trafficking, included forced prostitution and economic exploitation of girls and women (see Box 3.3).
- Violence against women in humanitarian and conflict settings.

The World Health Organization (WHO) definition of gender-based violence explicitly includes its impact: ' ... *[it] is likely to result in physical, sexual or mental harm or suffering to women ...*' As discussed later in the chapter and elsewhere in this book, the health impacts are substantial and often persistent.

Gender-based violence is best understood in terms of the ecological model presented in Figure 1.1, which highlights factors at all levels from the societal to the individual.

Globally, men are more likely to die violently and prematurely as a result of armed conflict, suicide or violence perpetrated by strangers, whereas women are more likely to die at the hands of someone close to them, on whom they are often economically dependent. In much of the world, prevailing attitudes justify, tolerate or condone violence against women, often stemming from traditional beliefs about women's subordination to men and men's entitlement to use violence to control women.

Prevalence in the UK

The Crime Survey for England and Wales (formally known as the British Crime Survey) is the most reliable source of community prevalence estimates of domestic violence and sexual violence in the UK. The 2011–12 survey reports lifetime partner abuse prevalence of 31% for women and 18% for men; 7 and 5% respectively had experienced abuse in the previous 12 months. The definition of partner abuse includes nonphysical abuse, threats, force, sexual assault or stalking. The Crime Survey for England and Wales also measures *nonpartner* domestic violence (termed 'family abuse'), reporting a lifetime prevalence of 9 and 7% for

---

ABC of Domestic and Sexual Violence, First Edition.
Edited by Susan Bewley and Jan Welch.
© 2014 John Wiley & Sons, Ltd. Published 2014 by John Wiley & Sons, Ltd.

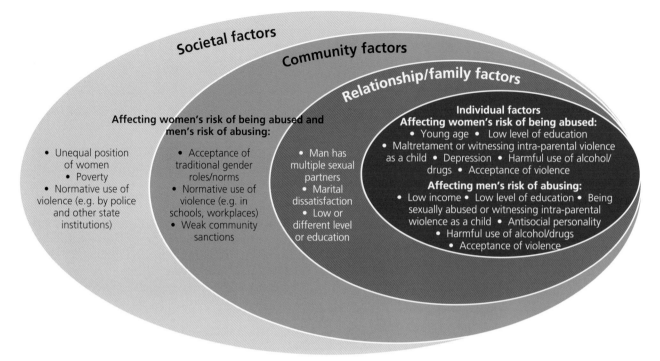

Figure 1.1 Factors associated with violence against women. Source: WHO 2012 Understanding and addressing violence against women: overview. Reproduced by permission of the World Health Organization.

women and men, respectively. The starkest gender difference in prevalence revealed by the Crime Survey for England and Wales is for sexual assault: 20 and 3% lifetime prevalence for women and men, respectively, although these figures include assaults by partners, ex-partners, family members or any other person. A more detailed examination of nature of physical abuse incidents recorded in 2001 also shows a greater gender asymmetry than the headline prevalence figures. Women, as compared to men, were more likely to sustain some form of physical or psychological injury as a result of the worst incident experienced since the age of 16 (75 vs 50% and 37 vs 10%, respectively), and more likely to experience severe injury such as broken bones (8 vs 2%) and severe bruising (21 vs 5%). Moreover, 89% of those reporting four or more incidents of domestic abuse were women. Data reported in 2010 showed that the majority of violent incidents against women are carried out by partners/ex-partners/family members (30%) or acquaintances (33%) rather than by strangers or as part of mugging incidents (24 and 19% respectively). In contrast, the majority of incidents against men are categorised as stranger victimisation or mugging (44 and 19%, respectively, vs 6% domestic and 32% acquaintance, mirroring the international data on murder discussed earlier).

The Crime Survey for England and Wales module on sexual assault reported that 2.5% of women and 0.4% of men aged 16–59 had experienced a sexual assault (including attempts) in the previous 12 months. It also showed that 0.6% of women and 0.1% of men had been the victim of a serious sexual assault in the year prior to interview. It did not distinguish between sexual violence as part of domestic violence and that perpetrated by a friend or stranger.

Domestic violence internationally

The WHO multicountry study conducted in 2000–03 estimated the extent of physical and sexual intimate partner violence against women in 15 sites across 10 countries (Bangladesh, Brazil, Ethiopia, Japan, Namibia, Peru, Samoa, Serbia and Montenegro, Tanzania and Thailand). This study, involving 24 000 participants aged 14–59 years and using standardised survey methods, is the most robust comparison between countries conducted to date, although figures do not represent national prevalence rates as the samples were based in specific rural or urban settings.

The reported lifetime prevalence of physical and/or sexual violence for ever-partnered women varied from 15 to 71%; 12-month prevalence rates varied from 4 to 54%. The percentage of ever-partnered women in the population who had experienced severe physical violence ranged from 4% in Japan (city) to 49% in Peru (province). The proportion of women reporting one or more acts of their partner's controlling behaviour (including isolation from family and friends and having to seek permission before seeking medical treatment) ranged from 21 to 90%. These wide-ranging rates may reflect cultural differences in the normative level of control in intimate relationships. However, the finding that women across all sites who suffered physical or sexual partner violence were substantially more likely to experience severe controlling behaviours compared to nonabused women concurs with the view that coercive control is a defining feature of interpersonal violence, irrespective of culture. Moreover, the WHO study revealed consistent health consequences supporting their reference to impact in the definition of interpersonal violence.

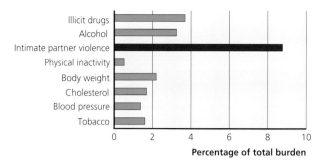

Figure 1.2 Top risk factors contributing to the disease burden in women aged 15–44 years in Victoria, Australia. Data from Vos *et al.* (2006).

Health impacts

Disease burden

The WHO multicountry study also measured health status, in order to assess the extent to which physical and sexual violence were associated with adverse health outcomes. The survey focused on general health and disabling symptoms, and found significant associations between lifetime experiences of interpersonal violence and self-reported poor health and specific health problems in the previous 4 weeks: difficulty walking, difficulty with daily activities, pain, memory loss, dizziness and vaginal discharge. The increased risk varied by symptom, ranging from 50 to 80%.

The first burden-of-disease analysis was conducted in Australia, reporting that interpersonal violence contributed 8% of the total disease burden in women aged 15–44 (3% in all women) and was the leading contributor to death, disability and illness for that age group, ahead of higher-profile risk factors such as diabetes, high blood pressure, smoking and obesity (see Figure 1.2).

Reproductive health problems

All studies of maternal mortality find that a substantial proportion of deaths result from assault by a partner. There are consistent findings of lower-birthweight babies for women who reported physical, sexual or emotional abuse during pregnancy. Other adverse pregnancy outcomes such as miscarriage and stillbirth may be associated with violence in pregnancy, although the associations are less consistent across studies. Gynaecological symptoms, sexually transmitted infections (STIs) and urinary tract infections (UTIs) are increased two- to threefold in women experiencing domestic and/or sexual violence (see Chapters 16 and 17).

Injuries

Injuries vary from minor abrasions to life-threatening trauma. While there can be overlap between injuries resulting from interpersonal violence and injuries from other causes, the former are more than 20-fold more likely to involve trauma to the head, face and neck. Multiple facial injuries are suggestive of interpersonal violence rather than other causes. The most specific for interpersonal violence include zygomatic complex fractures, orbital blow-out fractures and perforated tympanic membrane. Blunt-force trauma to the forearms should also raise suspicion of interpersonal violence, suggesting defence wounds (see Chapters 12 and 13).

Primary care

Common presenting complaints and chronic physical conditions are more likely in women who have experienced domestic violence (Box 1.1). In one US study, women who experienced intimate-partner violence after controlling for potential confounders such as age, race, income and childhood exposure to intimate-partner violence, had an increased risk of a wide range of debilitating complaints (see Chapters 3, 7 and 11).

Box 1.1 Women who experience intimate partner violence have increased risk of:

- Disability preventing work (1.5×).
- Chronic neck or back pain (1.5×).
- Chronic pelvic pain (1.5×).
- Arthritis (1.5×).
- Hearing loss (2×).
- Angina (2×).
- Bladder and kidney infections (2×).
- Stomach ulcers (2×).
- Sexually transmitted infections (STIs) (3×).
- Irritable bowel syndrome (IBS) (4×).

Mental health

The long-term mental health consequences of domestic and sexual violence overshadow the substantial impact of the physical health consequences (see Box 1.2). Systematic review of the (mostly) cross-sectional studies of women experiencing domestic violence show consistently raised risk of a wide range of mental health conditions (see Chapters 4 and 15).

Box 1.2 Women who experience domestic violence have increased risk of:

- Depressive disorder (3×).
- Anxiety disorder (4×).
- Alcohol and substance abuse (5×).
- Post-traumatic stress disorder (PTSD) (7×).

Experience of violence increases the likelihood of mental health problems (see Chapter 15), and it is also likely that people with these problems are more at risk of suffering domestic and sexual violence.

Intergenerational impact

Exposure to interpersonal violence during childhood and adolescence increases the risk of negative health outcomes across the lifespan. There is a moderate-to-strong association between children's exposure to interpersonal violence and internalising symptoms (e.g. anxiety, depression), externalising behaviours (e.g. aggression) and trauma symptoms. Children exposed to domestic violence are estimated to be two to four times more likely than children from nonviolent homes to exhibit clinically significant problems. Links are also demonstrated between children's exposure to violence and social development, academic attainment, engagement in risky health behaviours and physical health problems. While exposure to domestic violence undoubtedly represents a significant stressor in children's lives, studies indicate considerable variation in children's reactions and adaptations following exposure to this risky family context. Heterogeneity in children's adaptations is in part explained by the presence or absence of other adversities. Children exposed to domestic violence may also experience direct maltreatment, neglect, poverty, parental mental ill health, substance misuse and antisocial behaviour, which may compound the effect of exposure. The more adversities a child is exposed to, the greater the risk of negative outcomes (see Chapter 5).

Intersections with other adversity

The gendered nature of domestic and sexual violence reflects a power disparity between men and women globally. But gender is not the only social identity that makes people vulnerable to domestic violence. Disability, lesbian or gay sexual orientation, membership of an ethnic minority group, homelessness and uncertain migration status may increase vulnerability. There is uncertainty about whether the prevalence of violence is increased in these relatively marginalised groups. But there is growing evidence that it is even more difficult for individuals from these communities to disclose violence in health care settings and engage with domestic violence services post-disclosure. The intersection of class, ethnicity, sexuality and gender affects how domestic violence is experienced and how health care services respond. Any training of doctors and other health care professionals to ask about violence and respond appropriately needs to take into account the additional vulnerabilities of some patients who have experienced violence (see Chapter 2).

Epidemiological research

Although there are relatively robust estimates of the prevalence of domestic and sexual violence among heterosexual women, there are few studies of male victims or of men who have sex with men and women who have sex with women. With regard to health impact, we need more longitudinal studies if we are to understand vulnerability and protective factors. Such studies are particularly difficult to conduct, as are intervention trials with prolonged follow-up of participants, not least because victims of domestic and sexual violence often have difficult and disrupted lives. Yet if we are going to respond to their needs safely and effectively, this research is needed to guide the development of good practice and domestic violence-competent clinical services.

Further reading

Garcia-Moreno, C., Jansen, H.A., Ellsberg, M., Heise, L. & Watts, C.H. (2006) Prevalence of intimate partner violence: findings from the WHO multi-country study on women's health and domestic violence. *Lancet*, **368**(9543), 1260–1269.

Vos, T., Astbury, J., Piers, L.S., Magnus, A., Heenan, M., Stanley, L. & Webster, K. (2006) Measuring the impact of intimate partner violence on the health of women in Victoria, Australia. *Bulletin of the World Health Organization*, **84**(9), 739–744.

The World Bank (no date) Health and the role of the Health Sector, http://go.worldbank.org/C1UQRGBCE0 (last accessed 12 February 2014).

World Health Organization (no date) Gender-based violence, http://www.who.int/gender/violence/gbv/en/index.html.

World Health Organization (2012) Understanding and addressing violence against women: overview, http://www.who.int/reproductivehealth/topics/violence/vaw_series/en/index.html (last accessed 12 February 2014).

CHAPTER 2

'Culture' and Violence

Marai Larasi

Imkaan, UK

OVERVIEW

- Some manifestations of violence may disproportionately affect women and girls from particular social groups. Despite this, it is important that this violence is not defined simply as 'cultural'
- Generalisation and stereotyping risk losing the unique experiences, humanity and stories of individuals and marginalised groups
- The language and perception of *'culture'* are constantly changing; here the single quote marks and italics are used to say 'this is a loose term – use with care'
- By unpicking the everyday assumptions we all make, this chapter encourages a more nuanced approach to the subject of interpersonal violence for the health sector
- Doctors have a duty to work in the individual patient's best interest, so they must work to overcome their own prejudices as these may get in the way of accurate diagnosis and compassionate communication

What is *'culture'*?

'Culture' is perhaps one of the most contested notions within social, academic, human rights and even legal contexts. Yet *'culture'* has become increasingly important within public policy frameworks, impacting everything from health practice to criminal justice policies.

Work which seeks to understand and address violence against women and girls is no exception; *'culture'* is increasingly a part of how we think about *what* happens, to *whom* and *why*. Yet much of what we hear about the role and impact of *'culture'* (whether in conversations, the media or formal settings) problematises whole communities: the discussions build up the idea of whole groups of people as a 'problem' requiring a 'solution'. This may even risk further marginalising the very women and girls who need our support.

This chapter briefly challenges some of the 'common-sense' ideas around *'culture'* and the links between *'culture'* and violence against women and girls. It seeks to encourage health practitioners to adopt

ABC of Domestic and Sexual Violence, First Edition.
Edited by Susan Bewley and Jan Welch.
© 2014 John Wiley & Sons, Ltd. Published 2014 by John Wiley & Sons, Ltd.

a more careful and nuanced approach to how they consider *'culture'* in their work with women and girls.

Thinking about *'culture'*

In the UK, the term *'culture'* is often used in relation to peoples and communities who are considered to be *'other'*; that is, somehow different from that which is assumed to be the 'norm' and therefore authentically 'British'. In addition, there is often a conflation between ideas of 'race', 'ethnicity', 'community' and (increasingly) 'religion'. This inevitably results in the 'essentialising' of whole communities: the reduction of groups to simplistic, single elements. In practice, this means that men from some social groups are, for example, considered to be more (*'naturally'*) patriarchal and violent. Also, whole groups of women are viewed as more subservient and therefore more vulnerable. This can be easily demonstrated by a quick scan of much media reporting on forced marriage or 'honour-based' violence. Stories often focus on the 'cultural' issues rather than the widespread nature of all forms of violence against women and girls in all sectors of society. The effect is an echoing of historic, colonial perspectives that (re)presented some communities as less evolved. At the same time, individuals from black and minority ethnic (BME) communities may also use *'culture'* in a problematic way; for example, it may be a platform to promote ideas of an ideologically boundaried 'community' within which there is consensus around a range of norms and values.

The term *'culture'* is also used in the context of other 'groups'; for example, *'youth culture'*, *'gay culture'*, *'queer culture'* and *'gang culture'*. In each instance, the idea of *'culture'* suggests something fixed, established and clearly definable. Yet individuals from those 'groups' are likely to have a range of connections to, and understandings and interpretations of, that very same *'culture'*.

Given the difficulties that arise around the notion of *'culture'*, on the surface it might seem useful for practitioners to disregard *'culture'* altogether. Yet doing so would be equally problematic: *'culture'* is a significant factor in how we all live our lives (see Box 2.1). Therefore, it is a critical factor in work around violence against women and girls. What is important is that the perspectives we have described are challenged; otherwise, they might inhibit compassionate individual relationships in health care settings. For example, in order to begin to engage effectively with *'culture'* in this context we must avoid the conflation of *'culture'* and *'race'* in our thinking and assumptions, as these render some people as having *less* or *more* of any set of behaviours, attitudes and so on. We must rethink present notions that cultural identity is static, singular and one-dimensional. In reality, individuals often negotiate a range of different, interlocking and overlapping 'cultural' spaces with varying degrees of ease and tension, including family spaces, school and work settings, peer groups, youth or activity *'cultures'* and so on. We must come to terms with the idea that *'culture'* is dynamic and complex. While we can seek to understand perceived dominant norms and values, it is much more important to understand an individual's interpretation of, and relationship to, what is often described as *'culture'*. People are individuals and assumptions may inhibit good health care.

Box 2.1 **There are a large number of different dictionary definitions of 'culture'**

Social meanings

- The totality of socially transmitted behaviour patterns, arts, beliefs, institutions and all other products of human work and thought.
- These patterns, traits and products considered as the expression of a particular period, class, community or population.
- The predominating attitudes and behaviours that characterise the functioning of a group or organisation.

Abstract meanings

- These patterns, traits and products considered with respect to a particular category, such as a field, subject or mode of expression.
- Intellectual and artistic activity and the works produced by it.
- Development of the intellect through training or education, or enlightenment resulting from such training or education.
- A high degree of taste and refinement formed by special aesthetic and intellectual training and development.

Biological meanings

- The cultivation of soil, tillage.
- The breeding of animals or growing of plants, especially to produce improved stock.
- The growing of microorganisms, tissue cells or other living matter in a specially prepared nutrient medium.

Adapted from http://www.thefreedictionary.com/culture.

Thinking *'culture'* and violence against women and girls

The United Nations definition recognises violence against women and girls as both a cause and a consequence of women's unequal status in society, thereby acknowledging gender as the fundamental common point. However, the expression of that violence can (and sometimes does) differ depending on the social context in which a woman or girl is located. Women, girls, their families and their communities may describe or experience these contexts as 'cultural' (or not). This may have a major influence on their experiences, their help-seeking behaviours and their support needs. Some examples are given in this section.

Forced marriage

This often described as a purely *'cultural'* phenomenon, especially as it is much more prevalent in contexts where arranged marriage structures operate. However, women and girls may be forced into marriage in *any* context (e.g. pressure to marry due to pregnancy or to preserve premarital virginity). For example, during the conflict in Sierra Leone, a number of women and girls were forced to become 'bush brides' (being abducted by fighting factions, becoming 'wives' to combatants and thus being enslaved or providing and exchanging sexual and other labour to avoid destitution). Yet women who have survived this experience and are now living in the UK (legally as refugees or having been granted asylum, illegally or 'in limbo' while seeking asylum) are not routinely recognised as victims of forced marriage. Forced marriage continues to be viewed as a deeply rooted 'tradition' when instead it may often be related to civil war and a breakdown in societal relations (see Chapter 3, Box 3.2).

Urban violence/youth gang settings

These settings are sometimes described as having a *'culture'*: that is, a *'gang culture'*. While this is a matter of some argument, what is increasingly evident is that urban violence settings can often 'mimic' other conflict situations (such as insurgency or war) where sexual violence is used as a weapon. For example, a young woman who is associated with one youth gang, say as a sister or girlfriend, may be attacked by members of a rival gang as part of an ongoing territorial dispute. While the young woman might not approach the police, she may present at a genitourinary medicine clinic (see Chapter 16) or in the emergency department (see Chapter 12). A sensitive, well-informed practitioner may be the only option she has for a safe disclosure.

Humanitarian catastrophes

High levels of sexual and other violence are being increasingly documented in humanitarian situations. Women who have survived international or civil war, conflict, tsunami, famine or other humanitarian situations are likely to have been exposed to significant risk of gender-based violence. For example, women in refugee camps often describe routine sexual harassment and violence. Practitioners working with women who have survived conflict or humanitarian situations should be mindful of this when treating them for issues such as depression associated with their experiences.

Moving into practice

So what should health practitioners think about in relation to violence against women and girls and 'culture'? *Culture* has relevance in terms of both *assessing need* and *planning support*. It is important that practitioners are mindful that we all live within a *wider cultural context* where varying levels of violence against women and girls are tolerated and where many of the underlying structural causes of that violence are reinforced (e.g. gender inequality). But this should not be a 'tick box' exercise. As indicated in the example concerning forced marriage in the Sierra Leona conflict, an overemphasis on what is assumed to be cultural may limit engagement with women around their experiences.

Assessing need

At the point of assessing need, some key considerations should be:

- *How does the woman herself 'do' 'culture'?* That is, what are the norms and values that influence how she thinks, behaves and views the world and her experiences? For example, a woman may believe in the absolute sanctity of marriage. She may see this as important in terms of her *'culture'* and identity. This can have an impact on her help-seeking behaviour in that she may not feel able to disclose her experiences or to contemplate leaving a relationship.

- *Are there factors in the situation or context that have serious relevance?* For example, has the woman fled or lived through a humanitarian situation such as conflict or natural disaster? If this is the case then her risk of being exposed to violence (as well as the severity of violence) will have increased. Even as humanitarian situations begin to improve, many of the protective social structures that are eroded at times of societal upheaval will not be reformed immediately. In such situations, women often face increased risks of rape, sexual exploitation and other forms of violence. While requiring support with the direct consequences of her abuse, a woman or girl may be distrustful of authority figures, including health professionals. She may not feel able to discuss her experiences and may be fearful of and resistant to medical interventions.

- *How do the key figures in her life 'do' 'culture'?* The woman's relationship with *'culture'* may differ greatly from that of those around her, but they may use *'culture'* as an oppressive tool. For example, a woman from any social background may be committed to education and working outside of the home, but her male partner may believe that this goes against appropriate gender roles. He may use this as an excuse for abusive behaviour, citing *'culture'* as the reason for his abuse. What impact does this have on her safety?

Planning support

At the point of planning support (see Chapters 8 and 9), some key considerations should be:

- *Any immediate safety concerns*: The woman may need immediate access to a refuge, an outreach worker/independent domestic violence adviser or the police.

- *Avoiding making matters worse through inappropriate comments, behaviours or referrals*: Kindness, imagination, humility and an interest in other people and the diversity of human existence go a long way toward achieving best outcomes for the patient and thus good medical practice. But the development of compassion – an ability to see 'from another's perspective' and the facilitation of 'healing' (or empowerment, in the context of gender-based inequity) – also requires continual learning, challenging and reflecting on one's own norms and values.

- *Recognition of the complexity of and need for wider sources of support*: Where might the woman find allies, peers or ideological or religious support? Where might you find relevant information or specialist support organisations that have the understanding and networks to help (see Chapters 8 and 9 and Appendices A and B)? Throughout this book, examples are given of how violence and abuse might present in medical practice, along with 'clinical tips'

on how to improve one's practice. Many Black and Minority Ethnic (BME) women and girls prefer to access specialist BME-led women's services, but it should not be assumed that this is the case for all. Other groups, including young women, lesbians and bisexual and transgender women, may prefer specialist support (again, it should not be assumed that this is always the case). It is therefore important to find out whether there are specialist agencies that might be able to provide support and then whether this specialist support is important for the individual (see Appendix A).

- *Emotional support*: The woman might want to access emotional and therapeutic support. In this case, what she defines as *'culture'* may also be important to her. For example, a young, white, working-class woman from London may feel that it is important to speak with someone who is also from London with a similar class background, as this person may be able to relate to the nuances and key aspects of how she experiences and expresses what is often called *'working-class culture'*. Another woman from a black and minority ethnic *'community'*, not trusting the professional limitations of confidentiality, may not wish to see a nurse or interpreter who might possibly have a similar background in case they know people in common. This is important in understanding how she 'does' *'culture'* and what might be important to her in terms of support.

Box 2.2 **The 'one-chance' rule**

- If there is one chance to ask difficult questions and ensure the safety of a patient, it should be taken.
- Asking the 'difficult question' in a safe, confidential and sensitive manner may be the most effective way to determine whether a patient's relationship with her partner, guardian, relative or employer is coercive or dangerous or if she has suffered abuse in the past (see Chapters 3 and 7).
- Interaction with a health worker, especially during pregnancy, may be the only social interaction a woman has outside of a coercive relationship (within a sexual relationship, marriage or family) (see Chapter 16).
- It is important to always follow up by making contact with appropriate agencies that can provide counselling and advocacy and have the power ultimately to improve the woman's well being (see Chapters 8 and 9).
- Without making assumptions or judgements, responses and care should be tailored to the individual woman.

To maintain good record-keeping on patient safety, clinicians should ensure that:

- Concerns are only recorded in confidential notes accessible to other health care professionals but not directly to family members (see Chapter 20).
- Living situation details (i.e. with parents/partner) are recorded, as well as next of kin and partner details.
- Concerns are shared with appropriate professionals (e.g. the patient's GP) and relevant safeguarding teams are informed and involved (see Chapter 5).

Conclusion

Working with individuals from a range of different social backgrounds can be interesting and rewarding, but also daunting. It is crucial that health practitioners are able to recognise their own assumptions and biases and the impact these can have on their practice. The key is to maintain a fresh approach to each patient, remain alert to nonverbal signals and create individual space by having high standards of confidentiality (i.e. private time without third parties), so that good practice becomes your 'everyday' standard. Avoid accepting low standards as you will become jaded and miss opportunities to help. Be willing to ask the difficult questions (see Boxes 2.2 and 2.3), while avoiding the (very human) urge to stereotype whole groups of people; it is equally important that you do not ignore your concerns, as your questions and responses may help to keep patients safe!

Box 2.3 **Some suggestions for open-ended questions that start conversations**

- 'What does this mean to you?'
- 'How is this viewed in your [family/group/community]?'
- 'I understand there are a range of views about this even within your [community/religion/group], can you explain that to me?'
- 'I'm sorry I do not know much, but I'm concerned for you and wish to find out more.'

Further reading

van Gog, J. (2008) Coming back from the bush. Gender, youth and reintegration in northern Sierra Leone, ASC, http://www.ascleiden.nl/Pdf/asc9vanGog.pdf (last accessed 12 February 2014); winner of the African Studies Centre/Council for the Development of Social Science Research in Africa NiZa Africa Thesis Award 2007.

CHAPTER 3

Domestic Violence and Abuse

Fiona Duxbury

General Practice, Oxford, UK

OVERVIEW

- This chapter uses the Duluth model to help understand who is at risk of domestic violence and abuse (DVA), and why
- The chapter explores risk assessment, health impact and myths about DVA
- Research illustrates that DVA is an expression of a flawed relationship in that the exercise of power and control over another overrides mutual respect and compassion
- Anyone can experience DVA, but certain categories of individuals are at greater risk
- Experiences vary widely from mild to severe, even to death; two women per week are murdered in the UK by their partner or ex-partner

---

Box 3.1 **Home Office definition of domestic violence, 2012**

'Any incident of threatening behaviour, violence or abuse (psychological, physical, sexual, financial or emotional) between adults who are or have been intimate partners or family members, regardless of gender or sexuality. This includes issues of concern to black and minority ethnic communities such as so called "honour" based violence, female genital mutilation and forced marriage, and it is clear that victims are not confined to one gender or ethnic group.'

Gender

Although mens are also abused, generally there is a strong relationship between DVA and female gender. For the purposes of this chapter, the domestic violence perpetrator is referred to as 'he' and the DVA survivor as 'she', in order to distinguish between them and to reflect the more typical abuser/abused. The epidemiology of gender-based violence is covered in Chapter 1.

Teenagers

The Home Office recently amended the definition of domestic violence in light of recent discoveries of internal sex-trafficking rings in the UK and growing awareness of teenagers taking on adult roles both in partnerships and in having babies early. The new definition (Box 3.1) includes anyone aged 16 years or older, which may help to ensure that teenagers are not denied access to services for DVA survivors. While teenage survivors of DVA also come under child-protection legislation, they might not find help if they are independent of their parents.

Power and control: an explanatory psychosocial model

The power–control dynamic emerged as the key driver for perpetrators in qualitative research with DVA survivors carried out by the Duluth Programme in Minnesota, USA in the 1980s. The violence and nonviolence wheels (see Figure 3.1) derived from this research have since formed the basis of training on **R**ecognising, **R**esponding and **R**eferring those experiencing DVA in both the UK and the USA. Police witness statements from survivors and ongoing testimonies of abuse survivors have confirmed the validity of the model in practice.

The violence wheel's subcategories of behaviours, as described in the segments, might be updated to include harassment, humiliation and threat via social networks, text messages and the Internet, as well as same-sex relationships and woman-on-man DVA. The underlying dynamic of power and control remains, even if the form it takes might vary across genders and cultures.

Who is at risk?

Those most at risk of experiencing DVA are those with vulnerabilities. In short, bullies prefer the vulnerable because they are easier to control and isolate, giving them the sense of power they desire. Vulnerable groups in society are: women relative to men; the elderly; pregnant women; children; teenagers; the disabled; communities that are already discriminated against by others. The last include first-generation immigrants who do not speak English and those in same-sex relationships or transgender people. Already stigmatised, their isolation is greater, so revealing abusive

ABC of Domestic and Sexual Violence, First Edition.
Edited by Susan Bewley and Jan Welch.
© 2014 John Wiley & Sons, Ltd. Published 2014 by John Wiley & Sons, Ltd.

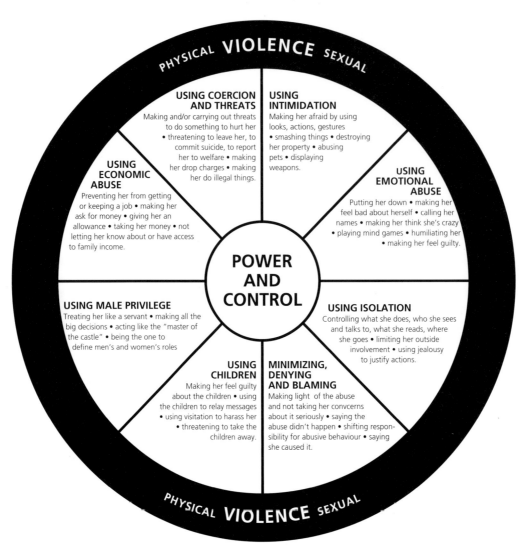

Figure 3.1 The Duluth model training wheel. 'The Power and Control Wheel was developed in Duluth by battered women who were attending education groups sponsored by the local women's shelter. The wheel is used in our Creating a Process of Change for Men Who Batter curriculum, and in groups of women who are battered, to name and inspire dialogue about tactics of abuse. While we recognize that there are women who use violence against men, and that there are men and women in same-sex relationships who use violence, this wheel is meant specifically to illustrate men's abusive behaviors toward women. The Equality Wheel was developed for use with the same groups.' http://www.theduluthmodel.org/training/wheels.html (last accessed 12 February 2014).

experiences is more difficult and more dangerous (see Chapters 7 and 9). Further discussion of 'cultural issues' is found in Chapter 2.

Women

The vast majority of DVA research remains focused on men as perpetrators and women and children as 'victims' or 'survivors'. The term 'survivors' is preferred to 'victims' because it indicates the active tenacity that those assailed must possess in order to survive daily and focuses on their strengths and assets. There is some justification for highlighting women as survivors, given that men are usually more physically powerful and the murder of women by men is much more common than vice versa. UK police audits have found that about 50% of murdered women are killed by a partner or former partner. Murder of men is more common overall, but it is much less often by their domestic partners. Women experience more sexual violence, more severe physical violence and more

coercive control from their partners and are more likely to be afraid of their partners. Sexual abuse is committed by men much more commonly than by women.

Pregnant women

A woman's physical vulnerability increases when she is pregnant (see Chapter 16). Indeed, one-third of women experiencing DVA are hit for the first time following impregnation. Those who become pregnant as teenagers are more likely than older women to be in an abusive relationship and also to have escaped DVA in their parental home.

Women at risk of so-called 'honour'-based violence and forced marriage

In so-called 'honour-based violence', the assertion of the power and control that resides in a strict, authoritarian, patriarchal culture becomes the family's role, rather than an individual's. This is carried out by members of the immediate or extended family, which may include women as well as men. A daughter may incur so-called 'shame' and 'dishonour' by behaving in ways that might seem usual to another culture's eyes. Sometimes just a rumour is enough to elicit an abusive reaction (e.g. coming home late, wearing 'inappropriate' make-up or clothing, having relationships outside the approved group, running away or refusing an arranged or forced marriage – see Box 3.2). Women who are immigrants and are isolated by language may be unaware of available support. UK law protects the individual, but she must first escape her community to access the protection the law affords. Absolute confidentiality is paramount if this is to be achieved safely.

Box 3.2 **Forced marriage**

- It is not possible to assume the quality of a private relationship from outward appearances or civil status/marriage.
- Forced marriage is distinct from arranged marriage, which may be organised by parents or marriage brokers with the consent of, or at the request of, the individual.
- A marriage is forced when one or both of the individuals do not (or, in the case of people with learning or physical disabilities, cannot) consent to the marriage and pressure or abuse is used to make them go through with it.
- Forced marriage is defined as a form of violence against women and girls in the UK and internationally. Men can also be affected by forced marriage, but women and girls are much more likely to be at risk of multiple and overlapping forms of violence within this context (e.g. sexual and domestic violence).
- Pressure may be applied in subtle ways over an extended period of time (e.g. framed within notions of being a 'good daughter' versus letting the family down or bringing it 'shame'). Victims may not always recognise what is happening to them.
- The pressure to marry can be physical (including threats, actual physical violence and sexual violence) or emotional and psychological. There might also be a financial factor, where wages are stolen or money is withheld.

Identifying factors to look out for during consultations include patients who:

- Are young in age but have a previous history of multiple pregnancies.
- Are always accompanied to appointments.
- Have a controlling partner, family member or carer who speaks for them.

Good medical practice includes:

- Observing behaviours and interactions between the patient and her partner/partner's family or carer (and not making assumptions about 'culture'; see Chapter 2) and asking other members of the team (e.g. receptionists, nurses, midwives) about what they observe.
- Being mindful that some patients' vulnerability may be increased by factors such as youth or lack of knowledge of or familiarity with 'the system'.

- Keeping the patient's best interests and safety in mind at all times.
- Contacting the Forced Marriage Unit at the Foreign Office for advice; they can help before or after at-risk girls disappear for example, during school holidays.

Same-sex relationships

The prevalence of violence between partners is similar in homosexual and heterosexual relationships, but there is a relative paucity of research data for the former. Lesbian, gay, bisexual and transgender patients may doubly fear disclosure of violence because it involves revealing their sexuality too. The sense of shame and bewilderment is often greater for gay men, because there is less recognition of the problem and there are fewer networks of support. Using gender-neutral language when asking about 'partners' increases the likelihood that a clinician will be told about same-sex violence.

Prostitutes and victims of human trafficking

Prostitution (see Box 3.3) is a taboo and stigmatised subject, but involves both men and women (many of whom have children to support). Among prostitutes there are high rates of previous adverse childhood experiences (violence, sexual abuse, neglect) and other vulnerabilities that arise in young adulthood, including problem alcohol and drug use, homelessness, mental health disorders and experiences of violence. Some prostitutes may have been victims of human trafficking (internal or from abroad – see Box 3.4) or have experienced sexual exploitation in young adulthood or within a gang.

Box 3.3 **Prostitution**

- It is not illegal to exchange sex for money but it is illegal to solicit, advertise or make profit from sex ('pimping').
- Prostitution is rarely taken up as a 'lifestyle choice' (the mythical 'Belle de Jour' or 'tart with a heart'), rather than for financial need or to clear debt.
- Prostitutes can work alone or with others, from the street, hotels, shop fronts, escort agencies, massage parlours or brothels.
- Prostitutes may service many clients per hour for long shifts (e.g. up to 40 a day).
- Prostitutes may be imprisoned by criminal gangs.
- Prostitutes are exposed to risks of sexually transmitted diseases, pregnancy, humiliation and violence.

How to ask a patient about prostitution

Be nonjudgemental and gently ask:

- 'Have you ever been involved in sex work?'
- 'Do you have any health concerns or worries about this?'
- 'Would you like any help with [your symptoms/ drug habit/ exiting the sex industry]?'

Box 3.4 **Human trafficking**

Definition (UN trafficking protocol, ratified by the UK and in force since 2009):

- The recruitment, transportation, transfer, harbouring or receipt of persons, by means of the threat or use of force or other forms of coercion, of abduction, of fraud, of deception, of the abuse of power or of a position of vulnerability or of the giving or receiving of payments or benefits to achieve the consent of a person having control over another person, for the purpose of exploitation. Exploitation shall include, at a minimum, the exploitation of the prostitution of others or other forms of sexual exploitation, forced labour or services, slavery or practices similar to slavery, servitude or the removal of organs.
- Women and children are trafficked globally in the UK, both within and from outside the country, for the purposes of sexual exploitation, domestic slavery, begging and organ donation.
- Domestic workers are trafficked and coerced by employers, forced to work long hours, are unpaid and often live in poor conditions, commonly subjected to sexual exploitation and physical violence.
- Human trafficking is a form of serious, international and organised crime.
- It also occurs in communities where trafficked people are hidden in private residences.

Indicators or 'red flags' might include:

- Not being left alone.
- Being accompanied by an older man or several men (who may claim to be a partner, husband or 'uncle').
- A maid or servant being accompanied by her employer.
- Looking frightened.
- Speaking poor English.

Children

Perpetrators of DVA will abuse not only their partner but often their children too, directly or as witnesses; in 30–60% of cases the perpetrator is also abusing children in the family. This may be sexual (i.e. paedophiles may also be perpetrators of DVA). There is an intergenerational effect, although it is not inevitable (and children may need reassurance about this), and it does not excuse conduct: perpetrators are more commonly survivors of abuse themselves than those in the general population (see Chapter 5).

Disabled children

A meta-analysis has revealed that children with disabilities are about two to three times more likely to suffer abuse than their peers with no disability (Jones *et al.*, 2012).

The impact of childhood abuse: a psychosocial cycle

Symptoms and signs presenting to health care

The impact of DVA on children depends on their age (see Chapter 5). Infants develop problems with insecure or chaotic 'attachment', which can lead to borderline personality disorder (BPD) in adult life. Children experiencing maltreatment (directly or as witnesses to DVA) from about 18 months onwards, with its attendant emotional abuse (fear and neglect), will additionally be at risk of developing post-traumatic stress disorder (PTSD), depression, poor self-care and, in the teenage years, self-harm, eating disorders and substance abuse. 'Externalising' behaviours involving antisocial, aggressive and criminal behaviour are common, as are 'internalising', depressed or anxiety-driven behaviours with low self-esteem and poor self-care.

These conditions often persist into adulthood for survivors of historic abuse. Many children are resilient, but unfortunately, the abused may tend to become abused again, sometimes appearing compelled to expose themselves to similar situations to those in which they were traumatised (perhaps related to an inability to negotiate boundaries that were breached while still developing). The 'externalisers' may feel compelled to become the dominator rather than the dominated in their adult life; the dynamic of control and power remains to the fore. Mutual respect, loving and kindness are not part of their way of life or in their vocabularies as adults, instead they. 'Do it to him before he does it to you'. These patterns are not inevitable, with only about one-third of child abuse survivors going this route. Where they do occur, they may lead survivors to seek or be referred for medical help. Some consequences are given in Figure 3.2.

Range of abusive behaviours

Definitions of violence

One problem for researchers is that a range of behaviours can be termed 'abusive'. Cross-sectional surveys of DVA prevalence therefore vary depending on the definitions used, the population surveyed, recognition by that population that their experiences fit the criteria used and the population's willingness to divulge information. The experience of DVA is common, and commoner in the health-seeking populations of doctors' waiting rooms. At a conservative estimate, DVA is relevant to about 1 in 10 of those women sitting in the GP's waiting room.

Narratives that alert the questioner to a high degree of risk

In the UK, the police and DVA support workers use an assessment tool based on CAADA-GP (Coordinated Action Against Domestic Abuse) toolkits (see Appendix B).

The CAADA-DASH (Coordinated Action Against Domestic Abuse & Domestic Abuse, Stalking and 'Honour'-Based Violence) risk identification checklists were drawn up after consultation with police and frontline agencies dealing with DVA survivors. Many of the questions overlap with categories described in Figure 3.1. Flags for high risk are related to the degree of possessiveness and obsession that the perpetrator demonstrates and to their knowledge of and access to weapons (e.g. ex-soldiers). Those who mistreat animals are also more likely to mistreat humans.

Periods of high risk occur when the perpetrator feels he is losing control, especially if the abused person is trying to end the relationship. Psychological techniques of threat and control are now brought into play, and the level of sexual and physical

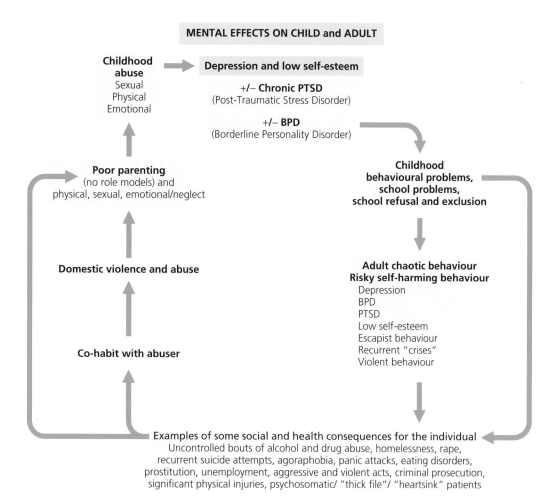

Figure 3.2 The psychosocial cycle of abuse. From Duxbury & Shakespeare (2000).

violence escalates. Sexual coercion, nonconsensual sex (or 'marital rape'), use of weapons, strangulation and threats to kill must all be taken extremely seriously as risk factors for murder.

Hearts and flowers

As time goes on, the degree of abuse usually increases in severity. This has been called the 'domestic violence hearts and flowers' cycle (see Figure 3.3). After an outburst of abusive behaviour, the perpetrator shows regret, brings flowers and claims undying love. There is a period of calm and reconciliation. Then the tension mounts again until the next outburst of violence/abuse. The abuse survivor still hopes that the relationship can be mended. She minimises the seriousness and blames herself, their circumstances or 'the drink'. Despite being unnerved, she agrees to try again. Each time this cycle goes around, the abuse meted out tends to get more severe. At some point the abuse survivor will describe a feeling of 'walking on eggshells' as the tension mounts. She may realise at this point that she is afraid of her partner, and that this cannot be described as 'love'. The level of risk in different abusive relationships can also vary unpredictably.

Teenagers, inexperienced in their first sexual relationships, may struggle to work out whether an abusive relationship might be an expression of romantic 'love'. Those raised in households without a norm of mutual respect in relationships may define relationships through the prism of power and control. The man must control, the woman must obey.

Perpetrators of DVA will not necessarily be obvious to associates and friends, and may appear charming to those outside the family. Some perpetrators may be privately ashamed of their behaviour but deny fault, blaming their partner or their circumstances instead. The myth that alcohol was the cause is used by perpetrator and survivor alike to explain away abusive behaviour. Rules of culture and religion may be used to justify behaviour that is not contingent upon that culture or religion (see Chapter 7).

Health impacts

Unsurprisingly, living in fear, danger and humiliation causes stress and health problems. These manifest themselves in attendances at GP surgeries, antenatal clinics, dentists' offices and almost every hospital department.

The role of the health worker is to *recognise*, *respond* and offer to *refer* patients who disclose DVA. To do this, the health worker must interview the abuse survivor alone (see Chapter 7). The perpetrator is most likely to be the one to have brought the survivor to the

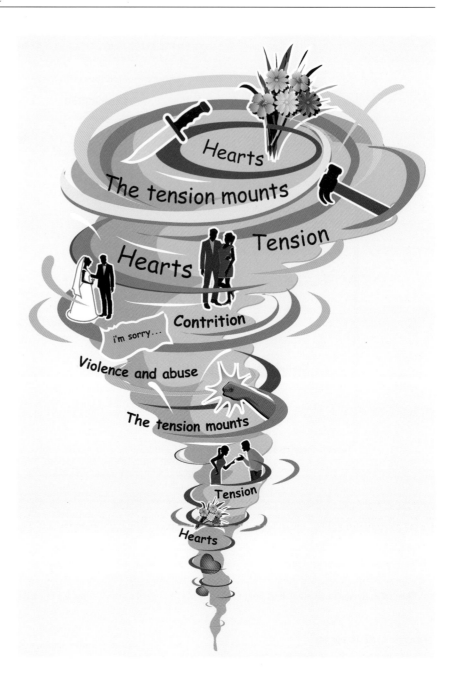

Figure 3.3 The 'hearts and flowers' downward spiral.

doctor's or the hospital. He does not want to be discovered and will appear concerned.

DVA is disproportionately common in populations that have: medically unexplained symptoms, chronic pelvic pain, recurrent urinary tract infections (UTIs), sexually transmitted diseases (STDs), poorly controlled asthma and diabetes, fibromyalgia, chronic fatigue, depression, PTSD, substance misuse, alcoholism or low self-esteem. The odds ratio for PTSD is seven times that in the nonabused population and shows a 'dose response': the worse the violence and abuse, the more likely the woman is to have PTSD. The odds ratio for gynaecological complaints is three times that in the nonabused population and also shows a 'dose response' to severity of DVA. There is an increased risk of gynaecological problems with a combination of physical and sexual abuse. DVA in pregnancy occurs in up to 20% of pregnancies and is associated with

intrauterine growth retardation, miscarriage, premature labour and postnatal depression. DVA is the commonest cause of injury in women between the ages of 16 and 60. Women who report DVA are over 30 times more likely to be afraid of their partner than women who do not.

The links between mind and body

Unsurprisingly, the DVA survivor, rightly fearing for her safety or life, may develop PTSD (see Chapter 4), which alters the allostasis of serotonin and glucocorticoids (see Figure 3.4). Decreased serotonin is associated with both depression and aggression. Cortisol affects brain development and immunity. The survivor may frequently attend surgeries or make but miss appointments. If living in fear, she may not concentrate well. Injuries to her mouth may result

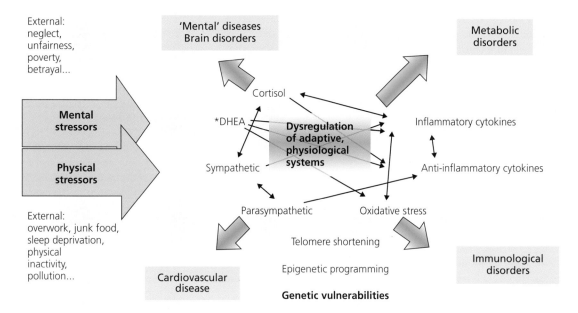

* Didehydroepiandrosterone

Figure 3.4 Protective and damaging effects of stress mediators: central role of the brain. From a lecture by Linn Getz, RCGP Conference, Liverpool 2011. Initial source: McEwen (2006). Reproduced with permission from Les Laboratoires Servier. Copyright © 2006, Les Laboratoires Servier.

in visits to the dentist (or dental phobia, as attending the dentist brings back the trauma). Avoiding DVA takes priority over other concerns. Regularly humiliated, she may become depressed, and her self-esteem suffers. She may not look after herself well. She may become the obese person who can never lose weight, who fails to exercise, who cannot stop smoking (even in pregnancy), who cannot look after her medication. The DVA survivor is more prone to diabetes/obesity, asthma and hypertension. Her unborn babies do not thrive. Her 'internal locus of control' is weak; she does not expect that she can control events but that events will control her. Nonconsensual sexual acts may result in recurrent UTIs and pelvic pain, and unplanned pregnancies. Her body and mind bear the scars. If she attends emergency departments, she may well present with injuries to the breasts, abdomen, genitals and face in particular, as well as fractures, particularly maxillo-facial, peri-orbital and skull fractures. She may have facial petechiae and marks of strangulation (which are difficult to inflict upon oneself) and bruises showing finger marks or from slaps/punches.

Her health will be less good than the norm for her population. She suffers from 'health inequality'. She may also find it difficult to work, and consequently be more likely than the nonabused to live in an area of deprivation.

Myths, fears and responses

Of the abused

The abused often feels to blame, particularly as her self-esteem is worn down by ongoing humiliation and put-downs. Not wanting to believe that DVA is the reality of her relationship, she tends to justify or minimise the abuse: thinking that she provoked the attack, that the children did not witness it, that it only occurred because he was drunk or under the influence of drugs. Another fear may be that protection will prove inadequate to prevent further abuse, should she contact an agency or involve other family members in trying to protect her. Statistics show that a woman is most likely to be severely beaten or killed as she tries to end an abusive relationship. If she reveals her abuse to anyone, she fears that events will spin out of her control. As her control over her life has already been eroded, any exacerbation is unwelcome. The final great fear, if she has children, is that they will be removed from her care. This is highly unlikely if she is trying to end the abusive relationship and works openly with professionals that become involved. Nevertheless, the UK Children's Act 1989 is clear that health workers and any agencies that hear of abuse must put children's needs first, over and above those of the parents.

Of the abuser

Most abusers delude themselves that the abused 'deserve' the punishment meted out (e.g. it was her fault for not having had dinner ready when he got home). Police questioning abusers often come across complete denial of acts for which there is robust evidence, such as CCTV footage or forensic material collected at the domestic crime scene.

The abuser fears being found out, so will nearly always threaten worse violence if the abused reveals their secret to anyone.

Some abusers do recognise their behaviour for what it is and want to change. Respect is starting to develop perpetrator rehabilitation programmes (see Chapter 10). However, where these programmes are run without accompanying protection for the abused parties, they can serve to make perpetrators more skilled at concealing their behaviour.

Of the health worker

Health workers often miss the opportunity to ask patients questions that might help in identifying DVA (see Chapter 7). It takes seconds to ask, or to hand out information. Although a disclosure may add 5 minutes to a standard consultation now, time is saved later. Considerable NHS time and money can be wasted on irrelevant attendances, investigations and procedures that miss the point.

Further reading

Bradford Hill, A. (1965) The environment and disease: association or causation? President's address to the newly founded Section of Occupational Medicine. *Proceedings of the Royal Society of Medicine.*

Campbell, J.C. (2002) Health consequences of intimate partner violence. *Lancet*, **359**(April 13), 1331–1336.

Carman, D. (2002) *No Ordinary Man: A Life of George Carman.* Hodder.

Duluth, P. (1984). Wheel gallery, http://www.theduluthmodel.org/training/wheels.html (last accessed 12 February 2014).

Duxbury, F. (2011) Violence against women and children. Royal College of General Practitioners e-learning Web site, http://elearning.rcgp.org.uk/.

Duxbury, F. & Shakespeare, J. (2000) *Consequences of Family Abuse Network Conference*, Oxford.

Golding, J. (1999) Intimate Partner Violence as a risk factor for mental disorders: a meta-analysis. *Journal of Family Violence*, **14**(2), 99–132.

Gerhardt, S. (2004) *Why Love Matters: How Affection Shapes a Baby's Brain.* Brunner-Routledge, Hove and New York.

Jones, L., Bellis, M.A., Wood, S., Hughes, K., McCoy, E., Eckley, L., Bates, G., Mikton, C., Shakespeare, T. & Officer, A. (2012) Prevalence and risk of violence against children with disabilities: a systematic review and meta-analysis of observational studies. *Lancet.*, **380**, 899–907.

McEwen, B.S. (2006) Protective and damaging effects of stress mediators: central role of the brain. *Dialogues in Clinical Neurosciences*, **8**, 367–381.

Van der Kolk, B., McFarlane, A.C. & Weisaeth, L.E. (1996) *Traumatic Stress: The Effects of Overwhelming Experience on Mind, Body, and Society.* Guilford Press, New York.

Widom, C.S. (1999) Posttraumatic stress disorder in abused and neglected children grown up. *American Journal of Psychiatry*, **156**(8), 1223–1229.

CHAPTER 4

The Impact of Trauma

Gwen Adshead

Forensic Psychiatry, Southern Health Foundation Trust, UK

OVERVIEW

- 60–70% of people will suffer a psychologically traumatic event in their lifetime
- The two most common traumas are traumatic bereavement followed by criminal victimisation
- Most people will experience psychological distress in the first 6–12 months, but only a third will experience chronic distress beyond this
- Psychological trauma reactions include post-traumatic stress disorder (PTSD) but also depression, anxiety states and substance misuse
- There are good-quality evidence-based psychological therapies that really help, and people should be referred quickly to trained therapists
- There is no good-quality evidence that telling people to forget about a trauma helps them recover or that PTSD is linked to compensation claims

What is a traumatic event?

There is nothing abnormal about feeling bad when bad things happen to you. But, as with fractured limbs, the fact that pain, distress and dysfunction are 'normal' does not mean that we do not intervene! Furthermore, over the last 30 years it has been recognised that traumatic events can lead to pathological stress reactions that, without treatment, cause severe distress and disability.

A 'trauma' or traumatic event is an experience that causes intense fear and helplessness in humans. Such events are usually (although not always) associated with imminent threat to life and serious injury. It has been known for centuries that people can still be affected for some time after they occur. Since the 1970s, post-traumatic psychological phenomena have been recognised as specific disorders that cause distress and dysfunction.

The commonest types of trauma are listed in Box 4.1. Doctors should be aware that medical interventions may also be experienced as traumatic and have been known to cause PTSD.

ABC of Domestic and Sexual Violence, First Edition.
Edited by Susan Bewley and Jan Welch.
© 2014 John Wiley & Sons, Ltd. Published 2014 by John Wiley & Sons, Ltd.

Box 4.1 Commonest types of trauma experienced

Commonest adult traumatic events

- Traumatic bereavement.
- Witnessing someone being badly injured or killed.
- Being involved in a fire, flood or natural disaster.
- Being involved in a life-threatening accident.
- Combat exposure.
- Physical assaults (men and women).
- Sexual assaults (women).

Commonest childhood traumatic events

- Sudden loss of a parent.
- Physical abuse (boys).
- Sexual abuse (boys and girls).

Does everyone who experiences trauma get PTSD?

Most people suffer a period of acute stress responses, which can last up to a year (Table 4.1). About 30% of people will develop longer-term post-traumatic conditions (PTSD, depression and anxiety states). It is important to try and prevent PTSD and other chronic conditions, because they are harder to treat once established.

Some people are particularly resilient (see Chapter 8) and seem to experience very little distress after trauma (possibly through genetic variation and other factors shown in Box 4.2). Other people are more at risk – usually those who have experienced childhood trauma or previous traumatic events. Some types of event cause more PTSD than others, such as events involving mass casualties and exposure to traumatic images, sounds and smells. Sexual assaults and violent crime cause more PTSD than noncriminal traumatic events (see Chapters 6, 18 and 19). Even a trauma of short duration may give rise to serious effects, although in general the more extended the trauma, the worse the effects.

What about the impact of childhood trauma?

Children who are exposed to frightening events may develop PTSD in the same way as adults. This is important to consider in children of refugees or migrants to the UK fleeing conflict and after events that affect whole families, such as road traffic accidents.

Table 4.1 Normal stress reactions after trauma.

Time period	Effects
Anticipation phase (often not present)	Anticipatory anxiety/fear, denial
Immediate	Shock, numbness, disbelief
	Acute distress
	Dissociation and denial
Short-term (1–6 weeks)	High levels of arousal
	Intrusive phenomena of trauma: thoughts, flashbacks, nightmares
	Poor concentration
	Disturbed sleep, appetite, libido
	Irritability
	Persistent fear and anxiety, especially when reminded of trauma: leads to avoidance behaviour
Long-term (6 weeks to 6 months)	Features described above persist, but should decrease in intensity and frequency
	Increased avoidance behaviour
	Irritability often most persistent
	Substance misuse (including alcohol) common as a way of managing arousal
12 months post-trauma	Possible anniversary reactions
	Persistent intrusive phenomena may indicate PTSD

Box 4.2 **Associations with development and maintenance of PTSD**

Risk factors for developing PTSD

- Magnitude and degree of exposure to the stressor.
- Gender (women have twice the rates of men, despite lower reported exposure).
- Previous personality traits, coping styles, experiences (a repressive coping style is protective: low anxiety and high defensiveness).
- Previous traumatisation.
- Peritraumatic dissociative experiences.
- Early sensitisation of the hypothalamic–pituitary axis.

Risk factors for maintenance of chronic PTSD

- Poor social support and organisational environment.
- Being divorced or widowed.
- Lower education and income.
- Concurrent family stressors.
- Low level of psychosocial functioning.

For some children, the traumatic events continue over months and years and are a cause of chronic fear and stress. The most common form of extended trauma in childhood is exposure to domestic violence and physical/sexual abuse. Between 10 and 20% of adults have experienced childhood trauma of this sort. This group is at increased risk of developing psychiatric disorders such as depression. Doctors need to be aware of the long-term effects of childhood trauma because there is good research evidence that exposure to childhood trauma increases the risk of developing PTSD after exposure to trauma in adulthood. There is also good evidence that childhood adversity increases health service utilisation in adulthood (see Chapter 5).

What are the signs and symptoms of PTSD?

The key features are:

- Re-experiencing phenomena (flashbacks, intrusive memories and images).
- Intense distress and anxiety.
- Phobic avoidance of anything that is a reminder of the event.
- Hyper-arousal or numbness.
- Intense feelings of anger or fear when exposed to reminders of the event.
- Disturbances of sleep, appetite and libido.

The neurophysiology is important to consider. People with PTSD have hypothalamic–pituitary axis dysfunction, resulting in persistent sympathetic hyper-arousal and disturbances of sleep and appetite.

Sufferers typically describe persistent mood disturbance, including numbness, rage, irritability, anger and fear. These mood disturbances have negative effects on social and marital relationships, leading to a lack of social support and isolation. They also are a risk factor for substance misuse (including alcohol).

Assessment

Some key questions for clinicians are set out in Box 4.3. It is important to bear in mind that the traumatic event may have taken place several months or even years previously. Pure PTSD is rare: comorbidity with clinical depression and substance misuse is extremely common.

Box 4.3 **Key questions in the assessment of post-traumatic disorders**

- 'When did the frightening experiences occur?'
- 'How long have you had symptoms?'
- 'How have you coped to date?'
- 'Are you using alcohol or other substances to cope?'
- 'What resources do you have to support you?'
- 'Have you had other frightening experiences in the past?'
- 'Have you seen a doctor for mental or psychological problems in the past?' (Previous traumatic history of psychiatric illness.)
- 'What was the traumatic experience you suffered?' (Criminal assaults or exposure to grotesque imagery are particularly 'risky'.)

In addition to classic features of PTSD, survivors of traumatic events may also experience persistent feelings of shame and (irrational) guilt. Identifying shame-based PTSD, as opposed to fear-based reactions, is important because treatment approaches are different.

It is better to ask about 'frightening experiences', as 'trauma', 'crime' and 'abuse' mean different things to different people. If the assessment is taking place in the context of an act of self harm then suicidal risk should be assessed for, even if the injury is minimal.

Poor outcomes are associated with a lack of social support and substance misuse. Poor outcomes are also associated with being dismissed or not believed by others.

Treatment

In the early period after a trauma (4 weeks), the best evidence suggests that 'watchful waiting' and general support is best practice. There is no evidence that one-off debriefing sessions are helpful in the treatment of PTSD, nor that they reduce the incidence of PTSD after trauma.

If a person is having PTSD symptoms at 4 weeks after trauma then treatment should be initiated to prevent the development of chronic disorders. Effective evidence-based treatments are available for PTSD. Treatment approaches for the post-traumatic disorders need to be comprehensive, flexible and geared to what the patient can tolerate. Box 4.4 shows the range of treatments available, the optimal types of therapy for different disorders and the timing of treatment.

Box 4.4 Indicated treatments for post-traumatic disorders

Acute stress responses

- Watchful waiting.
- Psycho-education and stress management.
- Social supports.
- Short-term pharmacological supports, e.g. hypnotics.
- Information and advice to families.

PTSD

If intrusive phenomena are prominent:

- Trauma-focused cognitive behaviour therapy (CBT) is the first line of treatment.

In addition/sequence:

- Eye-movement desensitisation and reprocessing; therapies need to focus on traumatic memories.
- Consider group therapy (psycho-educational or interpersonal) with other sufferers.
- Use selective serotonin reuptake inhibitors (SSRIs), especially where avoidance is prominent. Avoid benzodiazepines.

Treat comorbidities vigorously, especially depression and substance misuse.
Assess for suicide risk.

Patients with principally fear-based reactions need trauma-focused CBT that addresses the management of fear and anxiety. This uses techniques that focus on minimising intrusive and avoidance symptoms. Patients with shame-based reactions need a psychological therapy that focuses on cognitive representations of the self and relationships with others. Therapies must be trauma-focused. In addition to CBT, there is good evidence that eye-movement desensitisation and reprocessing is also helpful for the treatment of PTSD symptoms.

People with PTSD often struggle to engage with therapy, as it means thinking about something they fear, which is stressful and painful. Teaching stress-management techniques can be helpful in improving people's confidence and reducing avoidance.

Medication has an important role, both as symptomatic relief and directly in addressing pathology. Antidepressants, especially the serotonergic agents, may be helpful, as may tricyclics, because of their hypnotic effects. Medication alone is unlikely to be helpful, but it may be necessary to enable patients to undertake other types of therapy later, and it may enhance the efficacy of psychotherapy.

Group psychotherapy may be of particular use where the trauma occurs in a group context, such as in occupational settings or transport disasters.

What all doctors need to know

Normal recovery after trauma may take 6 months, or longer if there are further stressors. It is important not to be dismissive or judgemental.

The first sign of traumatic stress may be medically unexplained symptoms. Childhood trauma is present in a substantial subgroup of patients seeking treatment for chronic pelvic pain and other gynaecological conditions. In very anxious patients, it may be worth gently enquiring about experiences of trauma. Box 4.5 provides some further ideas.

Box 4.5 Thinking about the role of previous traumatic experiences in health settings

Ideas for role play or practice

1 A 16-year-old girl is complaining of persistent lower abdominal pain. You note that she presented to A&E two months ago after a small overdose and two cuts to her wrist, and that 12 months ago she was involved in an altercation in which a gang member was shot.
   What might be going on here?
2 An Irish woman in her 70s is referred for investigation of vaginal bleeding. She becomes agitated when you invite her to get on the couch so you can perform a vaginal and speculum examination. She seems dazed and confused, and initially fails to respond to command. You wonder if she may have early signs of dementia.
   What else might be going on?
3 A man repeatedly stabs his wife with a kitchen knife in front of their two children.
   Who is at risk of developing PTSD and other post-traumatic disorders?

Answers

1 This might well be a case of PTSD that has been missed because of the overdose. Antipathy by health professionals towards self-harming patients sometimes means that we do not explore the reasons for their behaviours. This might also be a shame-based PTSD, if she perceives the shooting to be her fault.
2 The patient may be dementing, but she may also be dissociating in response to a memory of sexual abuse. A substantial subgroup of the elderly Irish population, especially those who moved to the UK, were raised in children's homes where they were exposed to abuse and neglect of all forms. Culturally, and generationally, they may find this abuse difficult to talk about.
3 Obviously the woman (if she survives) and children are at risk; but consider also the extended family on both sides, both her parents and his. Police and emergency service personnel may be at risk and may need advice. The man himself may also develop PTSD for this event.

There is no evidence that patients benefit from being told to 'forget all about it' or 'put it out of your mind'. Intrusive phenomena that cannot be voluntarily excluded are characteristic of PTSD; patients are not actually capable of 'just forgetting'. Dismissal also gives the message to the patient that the health care professional does not want to hear or does not believe what they are being told.

Health care professionals may be affected by traumatic events. Doctors may be exposed to traumatic events for which their training has not prepared them. Be aware of the risks and take care of yourself and others. Every year, the General Medical Council (GMC) deals with cases of substance-misusing doctors whose problems probably began after exposure to traumatic events at work.

Further reading

Bisson, J. & Andrew, M. (2009) Psychological treatment of post traumatic stress disorder (PTSD), http://www.summaries.cochrane.org/CD003388 (last accessed 12 February 2014).

Centers for Disease Control and Prevention (no date) Adverse Childhood Experiences (ACE) Study, http://www.cdc.gov/ace/index.htm (last accessed 12 February 2014).

Ehlers, A. (2012) Post-traumatic stress disorder. In: *New Oxford Textbook of Psychiatry*. Oxford University Press, Oxford, p. 700.

NICE guidelines for treatment of PTSD in adults and children (2005), http://www.nice.org.uk/CG26 (last accessed 12 February 2014).

Stein, D.J., Ipser, J.C. & Seedat, S. (2009) Medication for post traumatic stress disorder, http://www.summaries.cochrane.org/CD002795 (last accessed 12 February 2014).

CHAPTER 5

Children

Andrea Goddard

Department of Paediatrics, Imperial College London, UK

OVERVIEW

- Domestic and sexual violence affects girls and boys, from infants to older teenagers, from all socioeconomic, cultural and ethnic groups, and occurs in all settings where children are found
- Some children are particularly vulnerable because of their circumstances, including disability, unstable home situations, families with mental health problems and/or substance abuse, homelessness, war, political strife and minority status
- Children with developmental disabilities are at greater risk, both as perpetrators and as victims. Unfortunately, appropriate prevention strategies are less readily available to them
- Domestic violence in the home is associated with an increased risk of physical violence against children
- Most sexual violence is perpetrated by someone known to the child or young person. Intimate partner (or teen dating) violence is increasingly recognised as a common problem in partnerships between young people. Those most at risk of stranger assault are adolescents emerging into the adult world
- Although domestic and sexual violence affect males, girls suffer considerably more sexual violence than boys. Their greater vulnerability to violence in many settings is related to gender-based power relations within society

Scope of the problem

Domestic and sexual violence occur in all settings in which children find themselves: home, school, neighbourhood, prisons, police stations and other forms of custody and detention, residential institutions and other forms of childcare outside the home.

Child sexual abuse and the sexual exploitation of children are forms of sexual violence. Both can take many different forms. Definitions vary by country and jurisdiction but there is always a power imbalance in the relationship between the abuser and the victim. Victims of sexual violence in childhood have an increased risk of adverse outcomes for health and well being in the short, medium and long term.

ABC of Domestic and Sexual Violence, First Edition.
Edited by Susan Bewley and Jan Welch.
© 2014 John Wiley & Sons, Ltd. Published 2014 by John Wiley & Sons, Ltd.

Domestic violence affects children and young people in a number of different ways. Children can be witnesses to violence between parents/carers in their family or perpetrators of violence in their own intimate relationships. Growing up in a household where there is domestic violence has well-recognised adverse effects on a child. Intimate partner (or teen dating) violence is increasingly recognised as a common problem in partnerships between young people.

It is important to note that the different forms of violence against children, including domestic and sexual violence, are not mutually exclusive but can overlap. Children frequently experience multiple forms of violence in multiple settings. Some children who experience violence in the family go on to become perpetrators of violence. Others become resilient and may even go on to be champions of campaigns against child abuse (see Box 5.1).

Box 5.1 **A child abuse survivor set up the National Association for People Abused as Children**

NAPAC (www.napac.org.uk) is a British nationwide organisation focused on supporting adults who have been abused in any way as children and who may never have discussed or received support for their experiences. The chief executive, who set up the organisation, was born and brought up in London. Painful memories of his childhood abuse kept coming to the front of his mind until, at the age of 38, he decided to set up a charity to help people like himself. NAPAC provides a helpline and a wide range of useful booklets, survivor stories and links to other Web sites and organisations.

Only a small proportion of acts of violence against children is reported and investigated, and few perpetrators are held to account. In many parts of the world there are no systems responsible for recording or thoroughly investigating reports of violence against children. Where official statistics based on reports of violence in the home and other settings exist, they dramatically underestimate the true magnitude of the problem.

Obtaining accurate data concerning sexual violence is often difficult, due to different definitions of what constitutes sexual abuse, underreporting, a focus on sexual abuse in specific settings and a paucity of any data in many countries. Most frequently-cited estimates of child sexual abuse have come from retrospective surveys of adults. Accurate information on sexual exploitation, female genital mutilation, forced marriage and honour-based violence is even harder to obtain.

Forms of sexual violence affecting children and young people

Child sexual abuse

The definition of child sexual abuse currently used in England is given in Box 5.2. It is similar to that used in other jurisdictions and by the World Health Organization.

> Box 5.2 **Definition of child sexual abuse**
>
> '*Sexual abuse involves forcing or enticing a child or young person to take part in sexual activities, not necessarily involving a high level of violence, whether or not the child is aware of what is happening. The activities may involve physical contact, include assault by pene- tration (for example rape or oral sex) or non-penetrative acts such as masturbation, kissing, rubbing and touching outside of clothing. They may also include noncontact activities, such as involving chil- dren in looking at, or in the production of, sexual images, watching sexual activities, encouraging children to behave in sexually inappro- priate ways, or grooming a child in preparation for abuse (including via the Internet). Sexual abuse is not solely perpetrated by adult males. Women can also commit acts of sexual abuse, as can other children.*'
>
> From: HM Government (2013).

From population-based studies in developed countries (Australia, New Zealand, Canada and the USA), it is estimated that the cumu- lative prevalence of any childhood sexual abuse is 15–30% for girls and 5–15% for boys ('any sexual abuse' includes noncontact, con- tact and penetrative abuse). For penetrative sexual abuse, estimates are 5–10% for girls and 1–5% for boys.

Most sexual crimes against children are not witnessed, and cases are unlikely to get to court (even in countries with adequate legal frameworks) unless the circumstances and physical evidence are overwhelming (see Box 5.3).

> Box 5.3 **Sexual predators may commit crimes against children with impunity**
>
> Within 3 months of the sexual abuse scandal involving TV presenter Jimmy Savile, some 589 people came forward with information, with a total of 450 complaints against Savile himself, mainly alleging sexual abuse. Early analysis showed that 82% of those coming for- ward reporting abuse were female, and 80% of the total victims were children or young people. Police said the number of sexual abuse allegations reported against a single person was 'unprecedented' in the UK, and 12 other inquiries or related reviews were launched. There has been a significant increase in the reporting of both 'nonre- cent' child abuse unrelated to Savile and previously undisclosed adult serious sexual offences. In London there was a fourfold increase in reports to the police's child abuse investigation teams.

Sexual exploitation

The sexual exploitation of children and young people under 18 involves exploitative situations, contexts and relationships where young people (or a third person or persons) receive 'something' (e.g. food, accommodation, drugs, alcohol, cigarettes, affection, gifts, money) as a result of performing, and/or others performing on them, sexual activities (HM Government, 2009). Child sexual exploitation can occur through the use of technology without a child's immediate recognition, via the Internet or mobile phones. In all cases, those exploiting the child or young person have power over them by virtue of their age, gender, intellect, physical strength and/or economic or other advantages. Violence, coercion and intimidation are common, as the child or young person's limited availability of choice results from their social, economic and/or emotional vulnerability.

Forced marriage

In many societies, a marriage or permanent union is arranged by parents and family elders, usually at or soon after puberty for girls. This occurs in some cultural groups and immigrant populations in mixed societies. Young people may be married in the country of residence or taken overseas.

Globally, the majority of countries have legislation which prohibits marriage of girls under the age of 16, and some forbid marriage under the age of 18. However, such laws are frequently ignored: marriages are not registered, customary or religious rules are accepted and few cases result in court proceedings even where clear legislation and statutory procedural guidance exist. Voluntary-sector organisations have been set up to help women and girls with this and other gender-based issues.

Early and forced marriage also directly impacts boys, on a smaller scale. It can have profound psychological consequences and is no less a violation of their rights.

Female genital mutilation

This is covered more fully in Chapter 17. Female genital mutilation or 'cutting' is seen by parents as beneficial – as a protection of virgin- ity, a beautification process and a precondition for marriage – but it has no medical benefit and entails an unacceptably high likelihood of pain and of immediate and long-term medical complications. It breaches international human rights laws, in particular the United Nations Convention on the Rights of the Child, and has been crim- inalised in much of the world. The UK is one of several countries that have enacted specific legislation in response to international migration of children for the purpose of procuring the procedure.

Infant male circumcision

There is controversy about infant male circumcision: views range from considering it a form of sexual violence and an abuse of the rights of the child to considering that the potential harm is slight and falls within the scope of parental freedom to determine religious and cultural rites for children. Circumcision is one of the commonest surgical procedures performed on males, despite there being few absolute medical indications. Worldwide, about 30% of men are circumcised, mostly in infancy; in most English-speaking and Muslim countries circumcised men form the majority. Opponents argue that infant circumcision can cause both physical and psychological harm. There is some contested evidence that circumcision is medically beneficial. Even if competently performed, it carries a small amount of risk, and most paediatricians will have seen cases with poor outcomes during their career. The rights and wrongs of this ancient practice are currently being vigorously debated both in medical journals and in some courts.

Forms of domestic violence affecting children and young people

Domestic violence from family members

'Domestic' or 'family' violence refers to physical, sexual, psychological or financial violence that takes place within an intimate or family-type relationship and that forms a pattern of coercive and controlling behaviour (see also Chapters 3, 7, 8 and 9). This can include forced marriage and so-called 'honour crimes'. Domestic violence may include a range of abusive behaviours, not all of which are inherently 'violent' in themselves or individually. There is mounting evidence that where there is violence between adults in the home there is also abuse of children. They may suffer and be harmed merely by witnessing the violence.

Intimate partner violence in adolescent relationships

A recent survey in the UK (Barter *et al.*, 2009) explored with young people their experiences of physical, emotional and sexual forms of violence in their partner relationships, with the following results:

- A quarter of girls and about a fifth of boys reported some form of physical partner violence.
- Nearly three-quarters of girls and half of boys reported some form of emotional partner violence.
- One in three girls and about one in six boys reported some form of sexual partner violence.
- Girls were more likely to say that the partner violence was experienced repeatedly.
- Family and peer violence were associated with increased susceptibility to all forms of partner violence.
- Having a same-sex partner was associated with increased incidence rates for all forms of partner violence.

Child perpetrators of sexual violence

Sexual behaviour as displayed by children and young people exists on a continuum from mutually agreed experimentation through to harmful, abusive exploitation. Retrospective research studies show that between 25 and 40% of all alleged sexual abuse involves young perpetrators. The majority of those are adolescent males, but young children and females also commit sexually harmful acts. Children and young people with learning disabilities are over-represented within this group but the reason for this is not fully understood. The majority of these children and young people have been or are being sexually, physically and/or emotionally abused themselves.

Adverse effects of sexual and domestic violence on children and young people

It is helpful to consider the harm that all forms of violence can have on children (see Table 5.1), as sexual violence usually overlaps with other forms of child maltreatment and is often associated with domestic or other forms of violence in the child's environment.

Management of sexual and domestic violence against children

Legislation on sexual violence against children, when it exists, varies widely. In the UK, a child under 13 years of age is deemed to be unable to consent to sexual acts, so both police and social

Table 5.1 Acute and long-term consequences of violence against children. Source: UNICEF (2006).

Physical health	• Abdominal/thoracic injuries • Brain injuries • Bruises and welts • Burns and scalds • Central nervous system injuries • Fractures • Lacerations and abrasions • Damage to the eyes • Disability
Sexual and reproductive	• Reproductive health problems • Sexual dysfunction • Sexually transmitted diseases, including HIV/AIDS • Unwanted pregnancy
Psychological	• Alcohol and drug abuse • Cognitive impairment • Criminal, violent and other risk-taking behaviours • Depression and anxiety • Developmental delays • Eating and sleep disorders • Feelings of shame and guilt • Hyperactivity • Poor relationships • Poor school performance • Poor self-esteem • Post-traumatic stress disorder • Psychosomatic disorders • Suicidal behaviour and self-harm
Other longer-term health	• Cancer • Chronic lung disease • Irritable bowel syndrome • Ischaemic heart disease • Liver disease • Reproductive health problems, such as infertility
Financial (direct, indirect and costs borne by criminal justice and other institutions)	• Treatment, visits to the hospital doctor and other health services • Lost productivity, disability, decreased quality of life and premature death • Expenditures related to apprehending and prosecuting offenders • Costs to social welfare organisations, costs associated with foster care, costs to the educational system • Costs to the employment sector arising from absenteeism and low productivity

services always need to be involved. Consent and confidentiality often present challenges in children aged over 13. Many do not want their parents informed and will refuse to involve the police or social services. Even when a young person is old enough to consent and has the capacity to do so, there remains a tension between their confidentiality and their welfare or that of other children. Always seek advice from senior local clinicians and child protection staff. Legal advice may also be required.

Medical management consists of psychological support and management of the risk of pregnancy and/or sexually transmitted infections. Ideally, management will be coordinated and undertaken by experienced sexual health, paediatric and child and adolescent mental health professionals.

Acute assault is defined by the likelihood of collecting forensic evidence – e.g. the sperm of the alleged perpetrator – and varies according to the gender and pubertal status of the victim:

- For all males and prepubertal girls, evidence can be collected up to and including 3 days after the assault (this varies by nature of assault; e.g. it is less likely that forensic evidence will be obtained from touching or kissing of genital areas than from penetrative rape with deposition of sperm).
- For post-pubertal girls, evidence can be collected up to and including 7 days after the assault.

Acute assault is best dealt with by a sexual assault referral centre (see Chapters 18 and 19), if available, as these are set up to deal with all aspects of acute assault and can maximise the collection of forensic evidence according to best practice (see Box 5.4).

Box 5.4 **Case study**

Case presentation

Mary Smith is a 10-year-old girl with mild learning difficulties. She lives with her mother Amy, who is a single parent, and attends mainstream school. Her teachers noted that she had been quiet and occasionally tearful for no clear reason in recent months. They tried repeatedly to ask Mary what the problem was but she would not say. The teachers observed that when Mary was picked up from school, Amy was sometimes accompanied by an adult male.

What else could Mary's teachers have done?

- Discussed their concerns with the school nurse and local Named Nurse for Safeguarding Children.

The general practitioner Dr Ahmed had not seen Mary for about 6 months. He saw Mary's mother about every 6 weeks for a variety of minor illnesses and menstrual problems, and had prescribed an antidepressant for anxiety and depression. Dr Ahmed had been concerned on two occasions when he noted Mary's mother had bruises around her eyes. On both occasions she claimed she had bumped into a door.

What could Mary's GP have done about his concerns of domestic violence?

- Discussed with a senior colleague or the Practice Lead for Safeguarding Children.

- Reported his concerns to the local Named GP or Designated Doctor for Safeguarding Children.
- Made contact with the local Domestic Violence Adviser.
- Mentioned a local domestic violence specialist service 'just in case' Amy or 'a friend' might need it.

One Monday morning at school Mary was really upset and crying. She eventually told her favourite teacher that her mother's boyfriend *'tried to put his willy in my bum'* on Saturday and that he had tried to do it several times before. *'I hate him 'cos he slapped my mum. I wish he'd go away and never come back.'*

The teacher immediately discussed Mary's disclosure with the school safeguarding children lead, who advised that they needed to inform Mary's mother and the local children's social services. They decided to discuss police involvement with the social worker. The duty and assessment team of the local children's social services responded promptly. A meeting between the social worker, Mary's mother Amy and the safeguarding lead took place at the school. Amy initially insisted, *'It can't be true. Mary's making it up because she resents me having a boyfriend'*. The social worker explained that she had needed to inform the police, who soon arrived at the school. A strategy meeting took place where it was agreed by the police and children's social care that it was in Mary's best interests that a full criminal investigation be carried out. Mary needed to be interviewed by the police and required a forensic examination. In England and Wales there is a recommended procedure for interviewing child witnesses known as an ABE (Achieving Best Evidence) interview, which is carried out by specially trained police and social workers.

Child forensic examination

Ideally the examination will take place in a sexual assault referral centre (SARC) with a specially trained paediatrician and/or a sexual offences examiner and child-friendly nurse or support worker. Children and adolescents should have the choice to have a parent/caretaker in the room with them for the physical examination, in order to provide support. The physical examination (including the anogenital examination) should be explained to the child/adolescent and parent in detail and consent should be obtained. The history of sexual abuse given by the child typically dictates the type of sexually transmitted infection (STI) testing necessary. Every child should have a complete head-to-toe physical examination, with a special inspection for any additional signs of trauma, such as bruising, abrasions or lacerations to the body beyond the anogenital region. Careful written and photographic (if possible) record should be made. The anogenital examination involves a thorough visualisation and inspection utilising an adequate light source. Photo documentation of injuries is advised in order to avoid repeated examinations. Sexual maturity should be noted. Less than 5% of children who give a history of sexual abuse will have a physical finding of concern for sexual abuse on anogenital examination. The ability of the forensic examination team to provide reassurance to the child and family that, despite what has happened, their body is normal – just the same as any other girl/boy – is crucial in helping them heal following sexual abuse. Where injuries are present, they can be reassured that healing will occur rapidly. Sometimes, however, it is useful to examine the child again a week or so later to document healing of injuries. Further information on these specialised examinations is available in specialised texts on this subject (see Royal College of Paediatrics and Child Health, 2008).

What happened next?

Mary and her mother were taken to a SARC. No evidence of abuse was found on physical examination or on examination of forensic material (body swabs and Mary's clothing and bedding). However, Mary gave a clear and detailed account of the episodes of sexual assault in an ABE interview. Her evidence was supported by accounts from her school teachers about Mary's disclosure of sexual abuse to them. The mother's boyfriend was charged with sexual assault but denied the allegations. Social services, working with the police, advised Mary's mother that unless she immediately ceased all contact with her boyfriend they would need to institute urgent care proceedings (civil proceedings in the family court). Child protection procedures were followed, culminating in Mary becoming subject to a Child Protection Plan. Mary's mother complied with the request to cease all contact with her boyfriend. Over the next weeks and months, support was provided to Mary and her mother by social services and the local child and adolescent mental health service, together with staff from Mary's school. Mary's mother subsequently revealed that the boyfriend had been very emotionally controlling of her. As the boyfriend worked as a swimming coach, his employer was contacted and advised of the allegation of child sexual abuse the day it came to police attention and he was suspended from his position while the inquiry proceeded. In view of the seriousness of the allegation, the Crown Prosecution Service took forward a prosecution, even though they judged there was a low chance of success. The charge was not upheld and the boyfriend was not convicted in the criminal court. He and his lawyer say he was falsely accused and are trying to get his job back. The case is ongoing.

Recognising and raising concerns about children in all settings

Children are looked after by their families, schools, communities and sometimes social care. In medical practice, it is not only general practice and paediatric services who see them – healthcare professionals in a number of specialities and healthcare settings may see children and young people who give rise to concerns about possible sexual violence. Just as when formulating diagnoses of medical diseases, doctors should be alert, have a 'low threshold for suspicion', develop skills and pattern recognition and recognise the value of training and asking for help when they are out of their depth (see Box 5.5).

Box 5.5 **Case study: children's needs may be relevant and identified in non-children's settings and clinics**

You are a junior doctor in a busy hospital outpatient clinic running late on a Friday morning in school term time. Your next patient has a reputation for being 'difficult', shouting at the receptionist and not attending appointments or taking her medication for her chronic disease. You notice she has brought a very quiet and ill-kempt 6-year-old with her, whom she has pushed roughly on to a chair.

What should you worry about?

1 Both the mother and the child.
2 The presenting chronic health problem.

3 Maternal mental health.
4 The child's welfare: physical (as unkempt), psychological (as withdrawn) and educational (as not attending school).
5 Hidden problems that may not have been identified (alcohol or substance abuse, violence, criminality).
6 Fragmented care.
7 Your own limitations (of time, empathy, knowledge).
8 Doing what is appropriate: we rarely address all of a patient's problems, but we may be able to demonstrate compassion, 'do no further harm' and alert someone who can help.

What should you do?

1 Be suspicious about the home circumstances both for the mother and the child.
2 In a complex case, your role as a junior doctor is to gather information, not to problem solve.
3 Try to develop a rapport with the patient and deal with her presented concerns.
4 Find out, *'How are things at home?'*, *'Who's at home?'* and *'Who supports you?'*
5 Make your 'usual enquiry' about social circumstances, smoking, alcohol, drugs, mental state.
6 Ask how the child is getting on: at school, are they passing developmental milestones?
7 Find out whether there are other children at home (number and ages) and who helps look after them.
8 Offer help: *'What can I do to help?'*, *'May I contact your [GP, health visitor, housing or social worker] to discuss your needs?'*
9 Do not challenge or get out of your depth.
10 Observe demeanour, but do not be fobbed off, whether by aggression or plausible, charming explanations.
11 Make a plan that addresses the mother's medical needs and follow up.
12 It is rarely urgent to take action in the here and now, but concerns must be followed up after the clinic.
13 Make careful documentation.
14 Discuss the case with a senior colleague.
15 Report your concerns to the safeguarding team at your hospital or practice, and also talk directly to the GP.

Further reading

Barter, C., McCarry, M., Berridge, D. & Evans, K. (2009) *Partner Exploitation and Violence in Teenage Intimate Relationships*. NSPCC, http://www.nspcc .org.uk/Inform/research/findings/partner_exploitation_and_violence _report_wdf70129.pdf and http://www.nspcc.org.uk/Inform/research /findings/partner_exploitation_and_violence_summary_wdf68093.pdf (last accessed 12 February 2014).

Crown Prosecution Service (no date) Safeguarding children as victims and witnesses, http://www.cps.gov.uk/legal/v_to_z/safeguarding_children_as _victims_and_witnesses/ (last accessed 12 February 2014).

Evans, S. (2012) German circumcision ban: is it a parent's right to choose? *BBC News*, Berlin 13 July, http://www.bbc.co.uk/news/magazine -18793842 (last accessed 12 February 2014).

Gilbert, R., Widom, C.S., Browne, K., Fergusson, D., Webb, E. & Janson, S. (2009) Burden and consequences of child maltreatment in high-income countries. *Lancet*, **373**(9657), 68–81.

Hinchley, G. (2007) Is infant male circumcision an abuse of the rights of the child? Yes. *BMJ*, **335**(7631), 1180.

HM Government (2009) *Safeguarding Children and Young People from Sexual Exploitation*, https://www.gov.uk/government/uploads/system/uploads/attachment_data/file/190252/00689-2009BKT-EN.pdf (last accessed 12 February 2014).

HM Government (2013) *Working Together to Safeguard Children: A Guide to Inter-Agency Working to Safeguard and Promote the Welfare of Children*, http://media.education.gov.uk/assets/files/pdf/w/working%20together.pdf (last accessed 12 February 2014).

Patrick, K. (2007) Is infant male circumcision an abuse of the rights of the child? No. *BMJ*, **335**(7631), 1181.

Royal College of Paediatrics and Child Health (2008) *The Physical Signs of Child Sexual Abuse: An Evidence-Based Review and Guidance for Best Practice*. Royal College of Paediatrics and Child Health, http://www.rcpch.ac.uk/csa (last accessed 12 February 2014).

UK Foreign & Commonwealth Office (no date) Female genital mutilation guidance, https://www.gov.uk/government/publications/female-genital-mutilation-guidelines (last accessed 12 February 2014).

UK Foreign & Commonwealth Office (no date) Forced marriage: information and practice guidelines for professionals protecting, advising and supporting victims, https://www.gov.uk/forced-marriage (last accessed 12 February 2014).

UNICEF (2006) *An End to Violence against Children: The World Report on Violence against Children*. UNICEF/HQ 05-1826, http://www.unicef.org/violencestudy/1.%20World%20Report%20on%20Violence%20against%20Children.pdf (last accessed 12 February 2014).

CHAPTER 6

Sexual Assault of Men and Boys

Michael King

Mental Health Sciences Unit, University College London Medical School, UK

OVERVIEW

- Sexual assault of men remains a taboo subject
- Men who are raped are often too embarrassed to speak about it
- Many people still do not believe it is possible to rape a man
- Many assaults are concealed and go unreported
- Doctors can respond well to men who are sexually assaulted

Definitions of rape and sexual assault

Men and boys who are raped experience many of the same difficulties that women regularly encountered 20 years ago when they reported rape. Furthermore, men are traditionally regarded as perpetrators rather than targets of rape and this stereotype is hard to break. However, since rape of men was legally recognised in England and Wales in the enactment of the Public Order and Criminal Justice Act 1994 and with subsequent changes in the Sexual Offences Act 2003, attitudes have changed.

Rape is now defined in law as an act wherein a man intentionally penetrates the vagina, anus or mouth of another person with his penis; when that person does not consent to the penetration; and when the man does not reasonably believe that the person consents. When penetration is with something other than a penis, the offence is assault by penetration. A woman can be charged with, or convicted of, rape as a secondary party, for example when she has helped a man who has raped another person. Other forms of male sexual assault by women are described by terms such as 'indecent assault'. Since the introduction of these wider legal definitions of rape, the police and medical services have become more familiar with how men who are raped should be assessed and managed.

Myths about male rape

At the outset, it is important to be aware of the many myths about sexual assault of men (see Box 6.1 and Figures 6.1 and 6.2). The first is that men cannot be forced to have sex against their will. It is assumed that men can defend themselves when threatened. In fact,

research has shown that people of either gender often feel helpless and submit to an assault due to panic and an overwhelming sense of disbelief. This 'freezing' is experienced by many men and women threatened with assault and may be a form of self-preservation in the face of a severe threat.

Box 6.1 Myth busters concerning sexual assault of men and boys

- Men can be forced to have sex against their will.
- Men who are sexually assaulted need not be gay.
- Men who sexually assault men are more likely to be heterosexual.
- Most gang rapes of men are perpetrated by heterosexual men.
- Sexual arousal can be involuntary and provoked by extreme fear or anxiety.
- Rape does not take away a man's masculinity.
- Rape does not make men homosexual.
- Female perpetrators are involved in half of sexual assaults on men and boys.
- Men may feel humiliated and that they should have been able to resist.

A second misunderstanding is that men who are sexually assaulted must be gay. This echoes earlier misconceptions that women who were raped wanted it or were in some way 'asking for it'. A closely related myth is that men who sexually assault

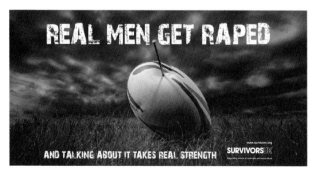

Figure 6.1 'Real Men Get Raped': education poster from self-help group SurvivorsUK. Source: www.survivorsuk.org (last accessed 12 February 2014). Reproduced with permission of Survivors UK.

ABC of Domestic and Sexual Violence, First Edition.
Edited by Susan Bewley and Jan Welch.
© 2014 John Wiley & Sons, Ltd. Published 2014 by John Wiley & Sons, Ltd.

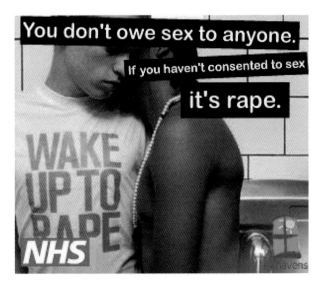

Figure 6.2 'You Don't Owe Sex to Anyone' Source: NHS image.

other men must be gay. In fact, evidence shows that stranger rape is more likely to be by heterosexual than homosexual men and that two-thirds of gang rapes are perpetrated by heterosexual men. A fourth myth is that if a man experiences an erection or ejaculates during an assault then he must have been complicit in some way. However, research has shown that extreme fear or anxiety in any situation can lead to erection and even ejaculation in men. Furthermore, erection and ejaculation are often involuntary responses to intimate sexual touching, particularly in a younger man, and are not an indication that he is sexually aroused. In fact, a perpetrator may intentionally stimulate the victim in order to arouse him, and this may make it seem that he wanted the assault.

Another assumption is that rape takes away a man's masculinity. An assailant may actually play on this possibility, given that rape is often an expression of power and control. For example, in war zones and other conflict situations, defeated soldiers may be raped primarily to humiliate and emasculate them. A further myth is that rape makes heterosexual men homosexual. Although confusion about sexual orientation is not uncommon in men following male-on-male sexual assault, there is no evidence that sexual assault affects a man's fundamental sexual orientation.

Finally, although it is commonly assumed that a woman cannot sexually assault a man, there is evidence that female perpetrators are involved in almost half of sexual assaults against men and boys. However, men's reactions to sexual molestation by women may be even more negative, because they feel strongly that they should have been able to defend themselves and resist the assault.

Response to the assault

While people who are sexually assaulted are always distressed by their experiences, their responses do not necessarily mean that they need immediate or specialist psychological treatment. Many men will come to terms with the assault by talking about the experience with someone who is empathetic, nonjudgemental and supportive.

Some men may have longer-term problems of anger, despair and anxiety and only disclose much later, to a sympathetic clinician who takes the time to explore sensitively what is troubling them. In some cases, they may develop post-traumatic stress disorder (PTSD; see Chapter 4).

Assessment of recent sexual assault of a man

The approach to a man who has been sexually assaulted follows the process outlined in Chapters 18 and 19, and is summarised in Box 6.2.

Box 6.2 What to do if a man or boy reports sexual assault

- Seek expert forensic medical opinion (for advice for yourself).
- Offer expert forensic medical examination (for the patient).
- If forensic medical examination is declined, take a detailed history and perform an unhurried, sensitive examination.
- Check if the patient would prefer a doctor of the same or different sex.
- Stop if distressed.
- Consider immediate HIV post-exposure prophylaxis and hepatitis B vaccination.
- Perform psychological assessment and offer help.
- Take baseline specimens as indicated.
- Make detailed records.
- Offer aftercare.

Assessment is best carried out by a sexual offences or forensic medical examiner in a specialist centre such as a sexual assault referral centre (SARC). It comprises a detailed history and systematic physical examination, looking for bodily injuries and trauma to the perineum, anus and genitals; samples may also be taken for forensic analysis. As most men are deeply upset after an assault, the assessment requires great sensitivity and understanding; ask about any preference for evaluation by a male or a female clinician (do not assume) and accommodate this if feasible.

The assessment should be carried out as soon as possible after the assault, but should not be rushed or imposed and must be conducted sensitively and carefully in order to avoid compounding the traumatic effects of the assault. A psychological evaluation should also be made, with the offer of subsequent psychosocial support. Assure the victim that the examination can be stopped at any time and remember that immediate medical needs take precedence over any forensic objectives.

The type of examination will also depend on how much time has elapsed since the man has sought help; after 3 days, DNA is unlikely to be retrieved from swabs but documentation of injuries may still be productive. Many men or boys who have been assaulted may have no sign of physical injury, particularly if they froze and consequently seemed compliant with the assault. Sometimes a man may not be certain of all the sexual acts that took place because of the effects of alcohol or drugs. In these cases (subject to consent), samples are best taken from all bodily orifices.

Detailed records should be kept of the entire medical history and findings, as outlined in Chapter 20. A case study concerning the sexual assault of a young man is given in Box 6.3.

Box 6.3 Case study: assaulted young man

You are a newly qualified doctor working in trauma and orthopaedics. A young man, Paul, is brought in by ambulance with the police following a severe physical assault by a group of young men. He is admitted with fractured ribs and a small pneumothorax. He asks, 'Can I talk about something which is worrying me?'

- *What might be worrying him?*

Paul's perspective

Not only did the youths beat him up physically, three of them also anally raped him. He is feeling upset and sore and is concerned about whether he has been injured inside, how and whether he will tell his girlfriend and whether he could have caught HIV.

- *He is not sure whether he can trust you in order to tell you what is worrying him.*

Things to consider

- *Privacy for the discussion that's been requested:* If Paul is in a curtained cubicle or on the open ward, can a private place be found for the interview?
- *Sensitive, open and non-judgemental questioning:* 'Would you like to tell me about what is troubling you?'
- *What are Paul's wishes:* Does he want to tell the police, be referred to a specialist centre and/or be examined?
- *Infection issues:* HIV post-exposure prophylaxis, hepatitis B vaccine, sexual health follow-up.
- *Follow-up:* If he does not want to attend a specialist centre, other sources of support.
- *Documentation*.

Learning points

Male rape frequently involves high levels of violence, weapons and multiple assailants. Victims are at significant risk of internal injury, HIV and later self-harm, including committing suicide.

Aftercare

Establish what sort of aftercare the man would prefer and/or needs, and arrange this where possible. At the very least (and given the man's consent), his GP should be involved, as he or she will be able to deal with subsequent physical complications of the assault and can be on the lookout for possible development of post-traumatic stress disorder (PTSD) in the man and psychological distress in his partner (see Chapter 4).

Arrangements should be made for follow-up, especially if HIV post-exposure prophylaxis has been initiated, and information should be provided about local sexual health services and sexual assault support services.

In terms of later, long-term medical presentations relating to previous sexual assault, see Chapters 4, 11 and 15.

What to do if the man does not report the assault

Many men and boys do not report sexual assaults out of a sense of shame, or because they blame themselves or do not recognise that what has happened is abusive. The latter view is more common where the perpetrator is a woman and where there may be stereotypical beliefs that any sexual attention from a woman cannot be seen as unwanted or abusive.

Doctors or other health professionals need to keep an open mind about the possibility of sexual assault, particularly when a man appears troubled by a recent sexual contact or is anxious about his sexual function. In discussing sexual matters, questions such as 'Have you ever had an unwelcome sexual experience?' or 'Have you ever had a sexual experience that you later regarded as unwelcome or just not right?' can be embedded in the conversation. Most men are happy to field with such questions and the professional will get an impression of whether or not the theme is of any interest. Even if he reports that no such thing has happened, this line of questioning allows the man to see that the idea can be discussed and gives him permission to return to it and possibly to have a franker conversation at a later time.

Further reading

Mezey, G.C. & King, M.B. (2000) *Male Victims of Sexual Assault*. Oxford University Press, Oxford.

Petrak, J. & Hedge, B. (2002) *The Trauma of Sexual Assault: Treatment, Prevention and Practice*. John Wiley & Sons, Chichester.

Abdullah-Khan, N. (2008) *Male Rape: The Emergence of a Social and Legal Issue*. Palgrave-McMillan, Basingstoke.

CHAPTER 7

Identifying Domestic Violence and Abuse

Alex Sohal[1] and Medina Johnson[2]

[1]Centre for Primary Care and Public Health, Queen Mary University of London, UK
[2]Next Link Domestic Abuse Services, University of Bristol, UK

OVERVIEW

- Health care professionals can identify domestic violence and abuse (DVA) given practical guidance on how to ask directly about it, stressing the use of language and specific questions
- Individuals who appear helpless and inactive may have complex reasons for their nondisclosure and perceived inertia
- The skills to respond compassionately and effectively can be acquired

---

How to ask about domestic violence and abuse

Identification is achieved by directly asking women whether they are experiencing domestic or sexual abuse, encouraging spontaneous disclosure or asking other health care professionals to consider the issue. Asking can be by selective enquiry (on the basis of presentation), routine enquiry (habitual social history) or screening (universal).

Ideally, professionals should be encouraged to ask women directly and to promote spontaneous disclosure only as part of a DVA protocol, with local specialist services and referral pathways identified. Recent UK guidance ensures safeguards are in place in general practice to protect safety and confidentiality (see CAADA, 2012). Boxes 7.1–7.3 describe how to ask, giving practical tips.

Box 7.1 How to ask about DVA

Ask safely

- Only ask when it is safe, when women are alone.
- Do not ask about DVA when women are accompanied by third parties, including friends and family members (who should not be used to translate): third parties can report back to a controlling partner and disclosure can precipitate further abuse.
- It may not be safe to ask all women.

Keep confidential

- Ensure that information on computer screens is not visible to third parties.
- Record DVA (if feasible, code on practice computer system).
- Understand local principles for guidance on information sharing (e.g. Caldicott Guardian principles in the UK), for example with the police.

Ask sensitively

- Use sensitively worded questions (examples are given later in the chapter).

Box 7.2 Case story: avoid compromising a woman's safety

A 43-year-old woman presented with her teenage son as translator. She had multiple symptoms, including shakiness, total body pain and a 3-day history of dysuria (no frequency or nocturia). She wanted antibiotics, which had helped before. The GP asked who lived at home and the son said that Dad had left as his parents are separating. The GP decided not to ask why, as it might have compromised the woman's safety if abuse was a factor.

The GP prescribed antibiotics for a possible urine infection. A follow-up appointment was suggested, including the urine culture result, using a professional advocate to interpret 'so that [the son] does not have to translate complicated medical information'. The woman and son agreed.

The following week, a double appointment was arranged with the professional translator present. The woman reported that she felt better but that abdominal pain persisted. The urine culture was negative. The GP asked why she was separating. The woman disclosed that her husband had been physically violent for many years and was addicted to drugs. The police had been involved and her children were aware.

At a third appointment, the GP asked about a previous contraception prescription. The woman said her husband occasionally returned and wanted sex. She was worried he was putting her at risk of sexually transmitted infections (STIs) and was surprised to learn that previous antibiotics would not have treated STIs. On further explanation, she was keen to be tested.

Lesson

Had the GP asked the son why his parents were separating, he might have reported that Dad hit Mum. As he still saw his father, he might

---

ABC of Domestic and Sexual Violence, First Edition.
Edited by Susan Bewley and Jan Welch.
© 2014 John Wiley & Sons, Ltd. Published 2014 by John Wiley & Sons, Ltd.

then have inadvertently mentioned the GP appointment and disclosure, which could have resulted in Dad challenging Mum or in another violent incident.

Box 7.3 **Case story: how confidentiality can be broken**

A 30-year-old woman confided that her new boyfriend did not like her going out with her colleagues. He had hit her after she got drunk at a work Christmas party, saying she needed to be taught a lesson. The GP recorded 'domestic violence experienced'.

A few years later, the couple, now married, attended together for travel vaccinations. The nurse brought up the wife's files on her computer screen, in view of the patients. The husband saw the entry on his wife's summary medical record. The wife could not believe that what she had told her GP in confidence had been passed on to her husband. The husband was furious about the accusation and made a formal complaint, demanding the entry be removed from his wife's notes.

What to ask

Once a DVA protocol is in place and it is safe to proceed, the subject can be broached using open questions and then further explored more directly (see Boxes 7.4 and 7.5). The open question, 'How are things at home?' invites the woman to talk unreservedly, preferably without interruption.

Box 7.4 **Initial questions**

- 'How are things at home?'
- 'Who lives at home with you?'
- 'Are things OK at home with your partner and family?'
- 'Are there any problems at home? Tell me about your relationship.'

The woman can curtail the discussion if she wishes. Most are expert at hiding, and will not reveal information until they have assessed your likely reaction. Women should never feel pressured into disclosing current or historic DVA.

Box 7.5 **Progressively more direct questions**

- 'Does anyone try to control you or what you do?'
- 'Are you ever humiliated by anyone?'
- 'Are you afraid of anyone at home?'
- 'Are you having any problems with your husband/partner/anyone at home?'
- 'Has someone hurt you?'

Why ask whether anyone tries to control the woman or what she does?

- 69% of women have reported controlling behaviour by their partner.

- The UK cross-government definition of DV now includes coercive control.
- This recognises the enormous impact of controlling behaviour (Box 7.6).

Box 7.6 **Patient testimony**

'There were several incidents of violence over the six years ... However, there were many more incidents of psychological and emotional abuse that went on even if there was no violence. These were about control and power and diminishing my self-esteem to the point of not being able to see what was going on or trust my own instincts.

'Because there were fewer incidents of violence, I didn't consider myself a victim of domestic violence. Only after the violence escalated, when divorce proceedings were started and my ex-husband started losing control over me, and the children witnessed the abuse, did I realise I was a victim and I must do something.

'If I had been more aware that I was suffering the psychological abuse and emotional abuse, I may have been more able to see what was going on and get the help I needed for me and the children much sooner.'

Source: http://www.bbc.co.uk/news/education-19640257 (last accessed 12 February 2014).

Why ask whether the woman is ever humiliated by anyone?

- Humiliation is defined as 'injuring dignity or self-respect'.
- Humiliation is plainer English, easier to understand and has more widespread usage than 'emotional abuse'.
- Emotional abuse alone can produce long-term adverse physical and mental health effects.
- Emotional abuse may have greater health impacts than physical violence.

Why ask whether the woman is afraid of anyone at home?

- Women who have reported DVA are 32 times more likely to be afraid of their partner than women who have not.
- Women who have ever been afraid of a partner have higher depressive symptom scores than women who have not.
- One-third of women reporting fear of a partner in the last 12 months have experienced severe combined physical, sexual and emotional abuse, 27% emotional abuse and/or harassment and 3% physical abuse alone.

The HARK questions (Box 7.7) are structured using a 'funnelling technique', starting with less direct questions and ending with more direct ones about physical and sexual violence. As well as facilitating disclosure, this structure emphasises the multiple dimensions of abuse: emotional, physical and sexual.

The HARK questions have been validated in a London primary care population and used internationally in research studies. In the UK, they are used in some sexual health and sexual assault services. They have been coded for installation on to many GP computer systems, with configuration of the HARK template as an electronic prompt triggered by specific conditions associated with DVA, such as headache (see Box 7.8).

Box 7.7 **HARK questions**

- **H**umiliation: Have you been humiliated or emotionally abused in other ways by your partner or your ex-partner?
- **A**fraid: Have you been afraid of your partner or ex-partner?
- **R**ape: Have you been raped or forced to have any kind of sexual activity by your partner or ex-partner?
- **K**ick: Have you been kicked, hit, slapped or otherwise physically hurt by your partner or ex-partner?

In the IRIS study (see Box 7.8), questions were not recited exactly; instead the template was used as a mnemonic, reminding the clinician to:

1 Lower their threshold to ask about DVA.
2 Ask about DVA.
3 Enquire about all abuse dimensions (emotional, sexual and physical).
4 Remember safety.

Box 7.8 **IRIS: the Identification and Referral to Improve Safety trial**

IRIS is the first European randomised controlled trial of a training support and referral intervention designed to improve the primary health care response to DVA and comprises:

- In-house evidence-based training for the practice team, on identifying DVA, appropriate responses, referral, recording, data handling, confidentiality and safety.
- Use of electronic pop-up prompts (HARK) in patients' medical records to remind professionals to ask about DVA.
- HARKS = Humiliate, Afraid, Rape, Kick and Safety ('Safety' is currently under consideration as an extra HARK criterion).
- Following a positive disclosure, asking whether it is safe for the woman to go home.
- An advocate educator from a specialist DVA organisation, who provides training and is the named contact for referrals. The advocate provides emotional and practical support, assesses risk, plans safety and signposts patients to other services.

Results

- Threefold increase in the identification of DVA.
- Sixfold increase in referral to specialist DVA advocacy services.

The IRIS model can be commissioned for practices; see www.irisdomesticviolence.org.uk (last accessed 12 February 2014).

In primary care, DVA is much more likely to present with ongoing health problems than an acute injury (see Box 7.9). Clinicians are therefore prompted to ask when women present with conditions associated with current or historic abuse, such as mental health problems (e.g. depression), medically unexplained symptoms (e.g. tiredness), gynaecological conditions (e.g. chronic pelvic pain) or chronic conditions (e.g. irritable bowel syndrome, IBS).

Box 7.9 **Case history: DVA presenting as health problems**

A 40-year-old woman consulted 14 times in the last year for problems including depression, dyspareunia and abdominal pain. She attended a routine appointment for a cervical smear and mentioned having an offensive vaginal discharge. In no consultation was she ever asked about domestic violence and abuse. Thus, she never disclosed that her husband criticises her looks and housework. He is physically violent when he feels that she is not keeping the house tidy. He expects frequent sex with her, which she does not enjoy. She feels guilty that she causes her husband to get upset. She says he is a great dad and well liked by her family and friends.

Other useful consultation questions aim to connect the woman's presentation with the underlying aetiology (Box 7.10).

Box 7.10 **Connecting questions**

- 'Some women with [these symptoms/this condition] may be at risk of suffering abuse from a partner or adult they live with. Is that happening to you?'
- 'Sometimes people with depression/low self-esteem have experienced major life events that cause this and which can explain why they feel so low. Living in an abusive relationship can cause this. Might that be happening to you?'
- 'Sometimes women with chronic pelvic pain have experienced other types of stress, pain or abuse in their lives, including sexual abuse. Has that ever affected you?'
- 'Sometimes people with chronic pain have a lot of stress or tension in their lives, which is reflected in their bodies. Might that be happening to you?'
- 'Sometimes the stress can be related to difficulties in a relationship. Some partners react strongly in arguments, using physical force. Is this happening to you?'

Questions linking symptoms or conditions with their possible aetiologies send out important messages about health impacts, as well as helping to identify DVA. They give women information that enables them to reframe their experiences and the effect on their health (e.g. Box 7.11). Even if women are not suffering abuse, posing such questions may indirectly help their friends and relatives who are.

Box 7.11 **Case history: how a woman reframed her abuse**

A 23-year-old woman saw her GP with low mood during the third trimester of pregnancy. She was referred to the perinatal mental health service. Postnatal depression was later diagnosed and antidepressants were started. Two months after the birth, she saw her GP, still with low mood but with good attachment to her baby and no suicidality. She admitted throwing away her antidepressants as 'they had not worked'. When asked about 'any problems at home, as sometimes depression can be caused by relationship difficulties?,' she described her poor marital relationship. Following a loving courtship, her husband stopped talking or listening to her once they were married. He went out with his friends and told her continually she was 'stupid, crazy and paranoid'. He convinced her that everything would be all right if they had a baby, but withdrew all physical affection when she conceived. He showed no interest in his daughter. The GP suggested that her husband's behaviour might have caused her symptoms. The woman replied, 'I knew that my problems would not be put right by tablets!' She was pleased that a doctor had confirmed that her low mood resulted from her relationship, not illness. The consultation then focused on the emotional abuse. Rather than helping her situation, the diagnosis of depression had allowed the husband's accusations that she was 'mental' and 'nuts' to gain ground. Her options were discussed. She felt this was a better use of time than further discussion about tablets.

Why 'state the obvious' about health impacts?

Why is it helpful to patients to tell them that sometimes people with depression, low self-esteem or other symptoms have experienced major life events that can explain their feelings, and that living in an abusive relationship can cause this?

- The health impacts may not be obvious to everyone.
- The patient may feel understood and safe to talk.
- Asking a direct question associating the clinical presentation with possible aetiology may be especially useful with mental health conditions.
- Physical violence causes adverse mental health outcomes, with a dose–response between the severity and duration of the violence and the prevalence of depression and post-traumatic stress disorder (PTSD; see Chapter 4).
- Mental health effects persevere even when violence has stopped.

Why state that sometimes women with chronic pelvic pain have experienced other types of stress, pain or abuse in their lives, including sexual abuse, and why ask whether that has ever affected the patient?

- The strong association between abuse and gynaecological conditions supports linking the clinical presentation to a possible underlying cause (see Chapter 16).
- Chronic pelvic pain and other gynaecological conditions (e.g. STIs, vaginal bleeding, genital irritation, dyspareunia and recurrent urinary tract infections (UTIs)) are more common in abused women.
- A dose–response has been demonstrated between combined sexual and physical abuse and gynaecological problems (three-times increased risk).

The last query in Box 7.10 shows how different questions may be used together. Flexibility helps the patient feel she is being treated as an individual. This engenders trust, increasing the likelihood of disclosure. Avoid reading standard questions from a computer screen; instead become adept at personalising the actual questions used in a consultation. This is best achieved through face-to-face training and practice.

The questions can have an impact regardless of whether the answer is positive or negative, as they signal that:

- DVA is an important health care issue and is unacceptable (contrary to what the perpetrator makes the woman believe, i.e. that it is her fault and is an acceptable reaction to her behaviour).
- Even living silently with DVA can affect the patient's health.
- The health care professional is prepared to listen and knows where to refer the patient for specialist support.

In general practice, disclosure is more often a process than a single event. Asking increases the likelihood that a woman will disclose at her own pace. Following disclosure of emotional abuse or physical violence, enquiry about sexual violence may be deferred to later consultations.

Reasons for nondisclosure

Women report wanting to be asked about DVA. Many will not spontaneously disclose unless directly asked. Despite being asked, answers may still be negative even if DVA has been experienced. The reasons for not disclosing overlap with those for apparent apathy in the face of offered help (see next section). They include:

- Personal perception of the abuse and its severity; believing that it is her fault.
- Shame, embarrassment and/or depression.
- Hoping for change while still feeling emotionally attached to the perpetrator.
- Using denial as a coping strategy.
- Being too scared to disclose at this particular time.
- Worrying that confidentiality will be breached (e.g. having heard receptionists chatting about patients at the front desk).
- Receiving threats from the perpetrator or other family members not to disclose.
- Concern that social services will get involved and that her child(ren) will be taken into care.

A woman may also decide not to disclose to an individual that she considers:

- A poor communicator or listener.
- Insensitive – not having offered privacy while taking the history or for the examination.
- Doesn't involve her in decision making, based on experience in this or other consultations.
- Doesn't respect her or care about her dignity (i.e. may cause further humiliation).
- Won't believe her.
- Judgmental, blaming her.
- Cold and indifferent.
- Unable to help.

Instead, the woman will wait to be asked by a compassionate person with whom she feels comfortable and relaxed.

Five practical tips on how to overcome barriers to disclosure

1 *Promote confidentiality as a core value of your workplace*: Train the whole practice team in the importance of confidentiality, in the reception area as well as the consulting rooms, and make it easy to provide feedback on lapses. Use the practice or service leaflet, web site and waiting room posters to publicise your team's maintenance of confidentiality and inform patients that they will be asked who is accompanying them and whether they want them in consultations.

2 *Explain social services' role in safeguarding children*: Social services' central role is to help parents protect their children, not to take them into care. The origin of a referral is not revealed to the perpetrator, and if the conflict escalates then assistance from statutory services will be easier to access. Extra support and scrutiny may serve as a warning, resulting in less conflict. Such information may be useful when enquiring about DVA and whether children are present in the household, and should be included in the service leaflet, web site and waiting room posters when the limits to confidentiality are explained (e.g. to prevent serious crime).

3 *Improve consulting skills*: Encourage health care professionals to sit in on each others' consultations in order to reciprocally feedback on listening and other consulting skills. Consider attending a consulting skills workshop.

4 *Encourage spontaneous disclosure*: Spontaneous disclosure is more likely once a woman feels that she can trust a service and that she will be listened to (Box 7.12).

5 *Ask other professionals*: DVA identification is often increased by talking to community-based staff with awareness of vulnerable families, such as health visitors, midwives, district nurses, school nurses and practice staff.

Box 7.12 **Spontaneous disclosure of emotional abuse**

Catherine is a 49-year-old disabled Caribbean woman with four adult children. Her GP practice is 'domestic violence aware'. Catherine saw a poster in the waiting room which prompted her to speak to her GP about domestic abuse. The GP referred her to a domestic violence advocate, whom Catherine met at the surgery. She spoke about her ongoing experiences with her husband, who had abused her verbally, emotionally and financially for over 26 years. Catherine had never told anyone before. She felt sad, low and unable to cope. The advocate provided practical support (with information and options for Catherine to consider) and consistent emotional support, and always discussed Catherine's safety. Catherine was seen for 12 months, initially fortnightly, then less frequently with supplemental phone calls and texts.

Over the year, Catherine remained with her husband and reported positive changes, including going out alone, leaving the house at least daily, meeting with a friend/family member weekly, opening her own bank account, taking a holiday to visit family, setting career goals and beginning a degree.

She reported 'having her life back' and 'feeling stronger to cope'. Her health and emotional well being improved, resulting in fewer visits to her GP and less medication for depression and sleeplessness.

Anonymised case study from the IRIS trial, www.irisdomesticviolence. org.uk (last accessed 12 February 2014).

Reasons for lack of overt action and helplessness in the face of offered help

Professionals should recognise their own negative feelings provoked by bearing witness to DVA. These may include:

- Helplessness on hearing painful experiences which you are unable to fix.
- Frustration when patients' choices are different from your own.
- Anger when children are exposed to DVA.
- Disillusion when a patient does not leave her situation, repeatedly returns to the perpetrator and seems unable to protect her children.

For the woman, decisions about staying and leaving are complex. Inevitably she has been made to feel that the violence and abuse are her fault. She believes she can stop it by changing her behaviour (e.g. by being a 'better wife') rather than by leaving. Living independently and safely may seem impossible from her present view. She is entangled in an emotional noose. She may already have received threats that she and her children will be harmed or killed if she leaves and evidence supports this: leaving an abusive relationship increases the risk of harm. The risk of serious physical assault or murder is higher at the point of separation and just after.

Women take multiple competing factors into account. There are the immediate potential losses of leaving: loss of love, trust, financial support, status, home (not having anywhere to go may include no recourse to public funds), family, friends and community (all of whom may take sides and blame the woman) and possibly work, as well as her children's loss of a father and/or school. The woman may depend on the perpetrator for alcohol and/or drugs. The perpetrator may be the carer for a woman with disabilities. Women from black, Asian and minority ethnic groups and those from lesbian, gay, bisexual and transgender communities may face additional barriers related to racism and discrimination. If the woman cannot speak English, she may face ongoing social seclusion.

Potential gains are long-term and less tangible: independence, autonomy, confidence, freedom, improved self-esteem and health for the woman and her children, not being abused and finding new, happy, intimate relationships. Women may have previous negative experiences of services, including not being believed (especially if the perpetrator is a member of 'the establishment', such as a police-officer, doctor or religious leader). Uncertainty about how change will affect her future means the instinctive choice is to stay put.

An example of an individual's weighing of losses and gains is shown in Figure 7.1. These may be finely balanced and will change with time, discussion, consideration of options, planning and the

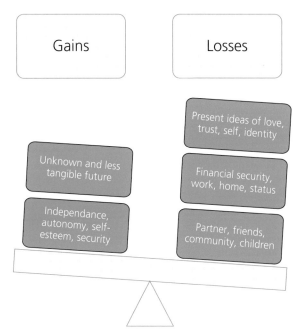

Figure 7.1 Initial weighing up of options for 'staying put', which may change with time.

emergence of self-worth. Information about options and respectful dialogue is key to constructive deliberation. Women may find it helpful to explicitly list such 'losses and gains', especially when advocates can identify those areas where practical support might make a difference.

Five more practical tips on how to get past barriers to perceived inertia

6 *Frequently tell the patient that it is not her fault*: Validate her experience regularly, not just on disclosure. Emphasise that the DVA is not her fault and that no one deserves to be treated this way. It is only when a woman begins to think that it is not her fault that she can become proactive (Box 7.13).

Box 7.13 **Possible validation statements if a woman discloses DVA**

- 'Everybody deserves to feel safe at home.'
- 'You don't deserve to be hit or hurt. It is not your fault.'
- 'I am concerned about your safety and well being.'
- 'You are not alone. Help is available.'
- 'You are not to blame. Abuse is common and happens in all kinds of relationships. It tends to continue.'
- 'Abuse can affect your health and that of your children in many ways.'

Reproduced from Hegarty *et al.* (2008).

---

7 *Support autonomous decision making*: You cannot judge all of the patient's considerations. Instead, your role is to help her balance contending factors, supporting autonomous decision making rather than deciding for her. Decisions conflicting with your own views should not be seen as a failure if they are thought through and regularly revisited as factors change.

8 *Decrease uncertainty*: Provide concrete advice; for example, abuse is a major risk factor for poor health. Offer a referral to a DVA advocate, preferably an appointment to be seen at the same premises. Inform the patient that the advocate will assess her risk and advise on how best to access safety, alternative housing, social care support, criminal justice and immigration advice. Do not make assumptions about whether or not a woman has recourse to public funds. She may be able to access benefits and public housing while applying for settlement under the 'domestic violence' rule. You cannot give immigration advice and should assist her in getting legal advice. A specialist DVA agency should be able to help her access this. Don't 'fortune tell' as the lifetime trajectory is unknown.

9 *Develop a long-term trusting relationship with the patient*: Continuity of care is paramount in helping women feel safe, encouraging disclosures and making frank discussion about the future easier. This may be impossible in some settings but is achievable in most health encounters (e.g. see Box 7.14).

10 *Organise face-to-face DVA training*: Evidence-based training and support programmes are available for whole practice teams. They include role play, simulated patients and case discussions within peer support groups.

Box 7.14 **Voices of survivors and clinicians from the IRIS research study (with proper permission from survivors and clinicians)**

Survivors' voices

- 'I told her. It was like we had finally found the piece of the jigsaw. The GP said that explains it … I mentioned about domestic violence … my GP acted on it straight away.'
- 'And you go to the doctors because you're feeling very unwell and they take your blood pressure and give you some blood pressure tablets and I thought, I've got to talk to somebody. And I said I don't sleep at all. Oh well, we'll give you some tablets for that and some tablets for this.'
- ' … the only doctor who ever asked … I was just so relieved that somebody just said something. And he gave me the box of tissues and I just sat and cried … and he said, tell me when you're ready, he said, there is somebody out there to help me. I'm not on my own. And if I want help, it's there and not to be ashamed of it. Which I was, really ashamed of it and he said, you're not on your own. We can get you this help. And he did. He really did.'

Clinicians' voices

- 'I'd known one of the patients who disclosed to me for 21 years. In that entire time I had no idea that she was living with a very controlling and psychologically abusive husband, and that this abuse played a key role in her health problems.'
- 'Since the training we have been able to pick up more cases and have been able to help women who had previously been unable to talk about their abuse. We are also more able to assess risk for the women and their children.'

Box 7.15 **What would make patients considering disclosure feel your practice is safe?**

- Waiting room leaflets, posters and signs in the toilets showing patients that you are aware of the issues.
- Awareness raising and provision of direct information to let patients know they are not alone and that you are interested.
- Provision of phone numbers and cards allowing patients to get help and bypass having to tell anyone if they don't want to share the information.
- An explanation of the importance of confidentiality in both the practice leaflet and posters in the waiting room.
- Trained reception staff wearing lapel badges stating, 'If anyone is hurting you, you can talk to me'.
- A 'domestic violence-aware' practice with congruence between the 'policy' and the 'practice' (i.e. 'we mean what we say') of all staff, from receptionists to GPs.
- Mechanisms whereby anyone can feed back good and poor practice.
- Staff confidence in the confidentiality and advocacy referral pathway.
- Implementation of the 10 tips given in this chapter.

Further reading

CAADA (Coordinated Action Against Domestic Abuse), in conjunction with RCGP and IRIS (2012) Responding to domestic abuse: guidance for general practices 2012, http://www.caada.org.uk/dvservices/CAADA_GP_guidance_manual_FINAL.pdf (last accessed 12 February 2014).

Feder, G., Davies, R.A., Baird, K., Dunne, D., Eldridge, S., Griffiths, C. & Sharp, D. (2011) Identification and Referral to Improve Safety (IRIS) of women experiencing domestic violence with a primary care training and support programme: a cluster randomised controlled trial. *Lancet*, **378**(9805), 1788–1795, doi:10.1016/S0140-6736(11)61179-3 (for further information, see: www.irisdomesticviolence.org.uk, last accessed 12 February 2014).

Fincken, C. (2012). Striking the balance: practical guidance on the application of Caldicott Guardian principles to domestic violence and MARACs, https://www.gov.uk/government/uploads/system/uploads/attachment_data/file/215064/dh_133594.pdf (last accessed 12 February 2014).

Garcia-Moreno, C., Jansen, H.A., Ellsberg, M., Heise, L. and Watts, C.H. (2006) Prevalence of intimate partner violence: findings from the WHO multi-country study on women's health and domestic violence. *Lancet*, **368**(9543), 1260–1269, doi:10.1016/S0140-6736(06)69523-8.

Golding, J.M. (1999) Intimate partner violence as a risk factor for mental disorders: a meta-analysis. *Journal of Family Violence*, **14**(2), 99–132, doi:10.1023/A:1022079418229.

Hegarty, K., Taft, A. & Feder, G. (2008) Violence between intimate partners: working with the whole family. *British Medical Journal*, **337**, a839, doi:10.1136/bmj.a839.

Royal College of General Practitioners (no date) e-learning course on violence against women and children. Reproduced from RCGP Online Learning Environment, http://elearning.rcgp.org.uk (last accessed 12 February 2014).

Sohal, H., Eldridge, S. & Feder, G. (2007) The sensitivity and specificity of four questions (HARK) to identify intimate partner violence: a diagnostic accuracy study in general practice. *BMC Family Practice*, **8**, 49, doi:10.1186/1471-2296-8-49.

Vos, T., Astbury, J., Piers, L.S., Magnus, A., Heenan, M., Stanley, L. & Webster, K. (2006) Measuring the impact of intimate partner violence on the health of women in Victoria, Australia. *Bulletin of the World Health Organization*, **84**(9), 739–744.

CHAPTER 8

Community-Based Responses to Domestic Violence

Nicole Biros

Victim Witness Advocacy, Boost Child Abuse Prevention and Intervention, Canada

---

OVERVIEW

- Domestic violence is a complex issue involving many sectors
- The language you use when enquiring about and responding to disclosures makes a difference
- Advocacy bridges the gaps that can exist between services and a survivor's needs
- The resilience of those experiencing domestic violence is central to their safety
- The safety of the survivor and her children must remain central to all responses
- Working in partnership will increase safety and save time
- Coordinated community partnerships decrease the risk of domestic violence

---

Background

Sadly, domestic violence happens more often and to many more people than we think. Fear – for personal safety, of the unexpected, of stigma and of much more – can be paralysing for someone experiencing domestic violence and can prevent disclosure to a professional. *Violence is never acceptable or excusable* and those experiencing it will need to hear this.

There are many reasons why women (and men) stay in abusive relationships. No matter what they are, those experiencing abuse are the experts in assessing their own safety and risk. Respecting this, and involving them in the process, will empower them to make healthy and lasting choices that improve their lives and help them exit the violent situation.

This chapter outlines the role and expertise of community agencies and the different forms of advocacy that they carry out (see also Chapter 9). It considers the language you should use when identifying and responding to disclosures and it looks at the strength and resilience of the survivors themselves, who must be involved in any effective response to domestic violence. This will be considered in relation to you, the health care professional, who will best

address domestic violence disclosures with effective partnerships and awareness of community work.

It is difficult to hear stories of pain and suffering and to know how to support someone in danger. With the right supports from expert community agencies, listening and responding to domestic violence disclosures can help to positively change a woman's life and those of her children. People working in health care can have a natural temptation to want to 'fix' the problems they encounter. However, domestic violence reaches beyond the realms of medical diagnoses and treatments and engages a community-integrated response. This chapter will shed some light on some appropriate methods of community partnership that you can utilise in your work.

The most important element in community-based approaches to domestic violence is to keep the survivor's safety central to any partnership or approach (see Figure 8.1).

Gender and language

Domestic violence can be experienced by anyone. It is important to acknowledge that the central features are power, control and fear. These are mostly endured by women, and they endure them more frequently than their male counterparts. For this reason, gender-specific language is used in this chapter, although the principles are similar for same-sex and female-to-male violence (see Chapter 6).

Advocacy

Advocacy on behalf of domestic violence survivors takes two forms: individual and strategic advocacy. The former looks at individual needs on a case-by-case basis and the latter considers the general political issues concerning large numbers of survivors. Most community agencies engage in both levels of advocacy, some focussing more in one area or the other.

Individual or personal advocacy

Advocacy is a key part of community work in the prevention of and response to domestic violence. Here, a woman is given a voice with which to express, request and receive appropriate care and responses to her needs. Research has found that intensive advocacy significantly reduces the risk of domestic violence, resulting in

ABC of Domestic and Sexual Violence, First Edition.
Edited by Susan Bewley and Jan Welch.
© 2014 John Wiley & Sons, Ltd. Published 2014 by John Wiley & Sons, Ltd.

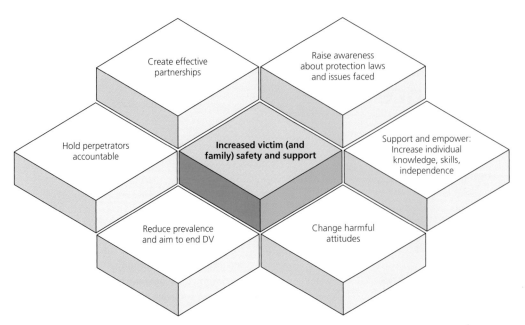

Figure 8.1 Model of community coordination with safety at the centre. Data from United Nations Coordinated Community Response Model, Centre to End Violence against Women and Girls, www.endvawnow.org (last accessed 12 February 2014).

67% of those who receive it remaining free of abuse (Howarth *et al.*, 2009).

Individual advocacy involves working directly with a survivor of domestic violence to make an effective plan of safety by accessing appropriate services and addressing individual needs (see Figure 8.2). An advocacy service can help to bridge the gap between

a survivor's needs and the varying services that may meet them. The individual issues and risks will be assessed by community agencies by reviewing with the individual her concerns, needs and desires for a future/safety plan. Community organisations specialising in domestic violence will engage with all of these services and coordinate their effective response to a survivor's needs based on

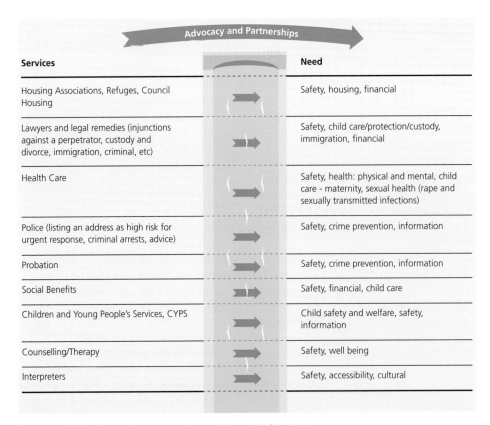

Figure 8.2 Examples of advocacy bridging the gap between services and the needs of survivors.

her plan of action. This is crucial to helping her to achieve the goals she sets out in a safe and expedient way, in an often chaotic and confusing web of services and procedures.

Advocacy is available to anyone experiencing domestic violence, regardless of their risk level. It is important to note that there are some services that provide service only to high-risk women. This is based on research into risk reduction. All stages of risk, however, are critical points of intervention, and low–medium risk levels can easily escalate.

Strategic/political advocacy

Strategic advocacy involves addressing broader issues of policy. It provides lasting improvements in policy and cross-sector partnerships that address issues of violence. Beyond engaging governments and responding to consultation papers, a community organisation will also engage local government bodies by offering training, attending meetings and linking into overall networking plans. This is done to improve other organisations' levels of awareness and understanding concerning domestic violence and to create professional links with those who will be in contact with the same clients.

Health care practitioners have the opportunity to form partnerships with the community. This is an excellent way of better understanding what community responses exist and how they might be engaged with when encountering domestic violence in their work. Preparation is critical; it is important to be equipped with suitable knowledge and tools before a crisis occurs.

Coordinated response: the practitioner and the community

As a sympathetic practitioner, you will receive disclosures of domestic violence. Being prepared with knowledge of the available services will significantly increase the safety and support you can offer. Inevitably, you will not have the time or skills to address all of a woman's needs and concerns, but knowing where to turn will ensure the best response.

The words, tone and body language you use when approaching the subject are critical in determining whether a woman will feel safe enough to disclose to you (see Boxes 8.1 and 8.2).

Box 8.1 **Sample prompts and responses to disclosures**

Prompts (more effective routinely than case-by-case)

- 'One in four women experiences domestic violence, and for this reason it is important to ask everyone if they are safe at home.'
- 'Do you feel safe?'
- 'Are you afraid of anyone?'
- 'These injuries are concerning. Is there anything you want to discuss about your safety? Is someone hurting you?'

Responses

- 'That must have been difficult to tell me. I am here to help.'
- 'Are you safe right now?'
- 'I believe you.'
- 'You are not alone.'
- 'I know of services that may be able to help and support you.'

Box 8.2 **Case study: learning from poor practice and feedback**

Nina Campbell was 34 years old and attending the hospital to give birth to her third child. It was normal, routine practice to ask pregnant women at 'booking' if they were experiencing domestic violence, even with no visible signs. The midwife thought that the booking question had been missed as it was left blank. She asked Nina, while she was still on the operating table following a caesarean birth, if she was in an abusive relationship. Nina was experiencing domestic violence but felt invaded by the way she was asked and chose not to disclose.

Challenges

- Inappropriate time and location.
- Lack of confidentiality.
- Nondisclosure prevents referrals being offered.
- Practitioner was nervous and did not know how to ask.
- Nina was not able to access available help.

Solutions

- Routinely ask patients at earlier stages.
- Awareness of safety concerns (training).
- Offer referrals anyway (e.g. 'You might have a friend who wants the information').
- Attend training and seek advice and support from local domestic violence organisations. Have information available in notes and posters.
- Involve survivors and the community in advice and helping to raise awareness.

Outcome

- Nina was given a discreet card with information for a domestic violence service before she left the postnatal ward.
- Three months later she got in touch with the domestic violence service. She began to make the courageous plan to leave the abusive relationship.
- She and her children are now safe.

Remember, this is probably not the first time the abuse and violence have happened. Even if the thought is terrifying or a shock to you as a professional, it is likely an ongoing trauma. This woman has probably developed coping mechanisms, including making light of her situation. Removing her coping strategies could be detrimental. The health care sector is an excellent point for intervention, as most members of the public will interact with it at some stage and caring and trustworthy people work within codes of confidentiality. What is most important to keep in mind is that no matter how you say it, provided you speak nonjudgmentally and kindly, you will be making a positive difference – for the future, if not now.

It is important to accept that it is not always possible to 'save' someone from domestic violence. This is a complex and deeply personal problem that demands a great deal of courage and strength from a survivor. It will require you to accept the survivor's choices and to support the move towards safety that she feels is best. This can be hard, because as professional 'helpers' we naturally want to act to preserve and save health, which is not always immediately possible with domestic violence. You may not see the end results of your positive actions, but remember how important your role is in the overall quest for safety.

Resilience of survivors

Those individuals who survive abuse can have an unconquerable amount of strength and wisdom. In addition to their ability to cope with terrifying situations, remove themselves from danger and begin their lives anew, they offer invaluable support to one another and important insight to professionals. See Box 8.3 for some advice on working with survivors.

Box 8.3 Considerations when working with a survivor of domestic violence

- Involve her in your response.
- Try to be creative with the resources that you have in order to ensure you can have some time alone with her to discuss her options.
- If you are making a referral to social services, involve her in the process.
- Note that calling the police is not always the best option; it can increase the risk in certain situations.
- Being judgemental decreases disclosure and increases risk.

Working with survivor-centred groups

Many organisations now involve survivors in their operational matters in order to ensure that the best approach and support are provided to others. As practitioners, you can work with survivor groups to gain valuable insight into best-practice models (Box 8.4) and how best to respond effectively and respectfully, as well as giving women the chance to gain strength and confidence through being recognised as experts.

Box 8.4 Best practice model

Mozaic Women's Well Being Project is an evaluated service within St Thomas' Hospital in London (www.mozaic.org.uk, last accessed 12 February 2014). Mozaic works closely with professionals in maternity and genitourinary medicine, providing training, consultation and specialised response to violence against women.

Routine enquiry in maternity and genitourinary medicine is accompanied by specialised training of health staff in how to ask about violence, respond appropriately and offer intervention via the Mozaic service integrated within the hospital.

Mozaic has a survivor-led charity and workshop series that involves survivors in the operation, planning and delivery of services in order to empower them and provide them with opportunities to develop skills and provide peer support.

This is an effective model of advocacy, bridging the gap between statutory and voluntary partnerships and keeping survivors of violence at the centre of the work.

At the very foundation of your work, what is most important is to remember that survivors will have insight into their situation that no one else can. Encouraging them to trust in themselves will increase their safety.

Box 8.5 Further practical issues after disclosure

Potential problems

- You do not have a confidential room in which to talk to women and ask about domestic violence.
- There is no interpreter available.
- A woman discloses domestic violence and says that she cannot go home as it is not safe.
- A woman has unstable immigration status and doesn't qualify for a refuge.
- A woman is asking for your help but is adamant that she does not want the police to be called as this will 'make things worse'.

Solutions to consider

- Who can you contact or engage?
- Are you able to ask the woman what she thinks is best?
- How would you assess her risk?
- How will you assess the safety of any children involved?
- Have you involved the woman in referral processes?
- What options are there, other than contacting the police?
- Be creative in your solutions.

Further practice is always beneficial. Try to attend training sessions that are offered and discuss issues with your peers.

Further reading

AVA Coordinated Community Response Model Online Toolkit (no date), www.ccrm.org.uk (last accessed 12 February 2014).

Bacchus, L.J., Bewley, S., Aston, G., Torres-Vitolas, C., Jordan, P. & Murray, S.F. (2010) Evaluation of a domestic violence intervention in UK maternity and sexual health services. *Reproductive Health Matters*, **18**, 147–157.

DIVERHSE Web site, http://diverhse.eu (last accessed 12 February 2014).

Hague, G., Mullender, A., Aris, R. & Dear, W. (2002) *Abused Women's Perspectives: The Responsiveness of Domestic Violence Provision and Interagency Initiatives*. ERSC, London.

Howarth, E., Stimpson, L., Barran, D. & Robinson, A. (2009) *Safety in Numbers: A Multi-Site Evaluation of Independent Domestic Violence Advisor Services*. The Henry Smith Charity, London.

Post, L., Klevens, J., Maxwell, C., Shelly, G. & Ingram, E. (2010) An examination of whether coordinated community responses affect intimate partner violence. *Journal of Interpersonal Violence*, **25**(1), 75–93.

Victim Services and Crime Prevention Division, Ministry of Public Safety and Solicitor General, Canada (2010) *Domestic Violence Response: A Community Framework for Maximizing Women's Safety*, www.pssg.gov.bc.ca (last accessed 12 February 2014).

CHAPTER 9

Sources of Referral and Support for Domestic Violence

Jackie Barron

Women's Aid Federation of England, UK

OVERVIEW

- All health professionals should be able to respond to victims and survivors of domestic violence
- There are a range of supports available in the community
- Ensure that you see the victim on her own, attend to her immediate health needs (e.g. if she has an injury) and assess any immediate risk to safety
- Give her time to talk and believe what she says
- Offer contact numbers for local and national domestic and sexual violence services but do not insist she takes any information in writing: it may not be safe for her
- Do *not* give advice – but support her in whatever decision she makes
- Keep detailed records in a safe place
- Ask how you and other agencies can get in touch with her safely in the future

---

What this chapter covers

- Safety and assessment of risk.
- An overview of specialist support services.
- Multi-agency risk assessment conferences (MARACs): what they do and when to refer.
- The role of independent domestic violence advisors (IDVAs) and specialist domestic violence courts (SDVCs).
- Domestic homicide reviews.

If a health care professional identifies or suspects domestic violence, or if a disclosure is made, this must be acted upon quickly and appropriately. The abuse may be current and ongoing or it may have taken place in the past. In either case, the survivor should be given a sympathetic hearing and pointed to suitable sources of help and support.

In most cases, giving contact details ('signposting') or directly referring to a specialist domestic violence organisation within the voluntary sector will be the first choice. Such organisations provide a variety of services, including refuge accommodation and associated support, advocacy, outreach work, counselling, support groups and so on. Many will also provide support for the survivor's children. They will be able to refer survivors to other services as needed, and will support them through practical and legal issues, such as getting rehoused or going to court (see later).

Remember that a patient will not necessarily disclose domestic abuse – or not on the first occasion she is asked. Health professionals should bear in mind the need to make routine and selective enquiries about abuse on a number of occasions, particularly when patients attend frequently with suspicious symptoms.

Box 9.1 **Case study: Janet Smith**

Janet was in an abusive relationship for 6 years, including physical, psychological and sexual abuse. However, she never discussed this with anyone. She was asked about domestic abuse when she was pregnant with her 3-year-old child, as part of a routine set of questions, but did not feel able to disclose it at that stage. The abuse usually took place late at night when her partner came back from their local pub. This led to Janet losing sleep. She went to her GP to ask for sleeping tablets but they didn't help much. She visited her GP a second time and told him there were times when she found herself crying for no apparent reason. This time, she was prescribed antidepressants. Janet visited her GP for a third time, feeling desperate and worried that she might be pregnant again. She couldn't bear the thought of having another child as she felt drained of energy, low and useless as a mother. When the pregnancy test proved positive, she asked for an abortion.

Safety and assessment of risk

If you suspect abuse, and the patient is accompanied by someone else, always ensure that you find a safe way to talk to her alone. Chapters 3 and 7 describe how enquiries about such sensitive subjects may be undertaken safely and explain the limits of confidentiality. If a patient discloses that she is currently experiencing domestic violence, it is crucial that any action you or anyone else takes does not in any way increase the danger she is facing. Your response to this disclosure could be crucial to her safety, health and well being, both now and in the future.

ABC of Domestic and Sexual Violence, First Edition.
Edited by Susan Bewley and Jan Welch.
© 2014 John Wiley & Sons, Ltd. Published 2014 by John Wiley & Sons, Ltd.

If a patient discloses abuse – however unlikely the story might seem – you must believe her, and show that you believe her. It is also important to be supportive and nonjudgmental. Case studies drawn from real life are given throughout this chapter (see Box 9.1).

The following actions should then be taken:

- Attend to her immediate health needs (e.g. if she has an injury).
- Assess the level of risk and ensure safety (see later). This will include:
  - assessing whether she or any of her children are at risk of immediate harm;
  - helping her develop a safety plan; or, if necessary, referring her to someone else who can help her with this.
- Give her time to talk, if she wants; or suggest someone else she could talk to.
- Give contact numbers for local and national domestic violence support services – perhaps by providing small cards – but do not insist she takes any information in writing: it may not be safe for her.
- Do *not* give advice on what she should do: it is her decision.
- Support her in whatever decision she makes.
- Keep detailed records, separate from the main patient record. Always ensure that these records can only be seen by those directly involved in the patient's care and that they are kept according to your Trust's guidelines on confidentiality.

Depending on your role, and the policies and procedures of your institution, some of the preceding actions might be undertaken by or in association with other health care professionals within your practice or hospital. If you do need to refer the patient to another member of your team, you should ideally ask her permission before you do so as this demonstrates respect and trustworthiness and enables her to feel in control.

Following on from this, and particularly where abuse is ongoing, you should make sure that any communications or actions will not alert the alleged perpetrator, unless or until the survivor wishes to do so. Ask her how you can get in touch with her safely in future, should you need to. If you have to give her details to another agency, for example because of child protection issues, ensure that they also know how they can contact her safely.

Ideally, a risk assessment should be undertaken with anyone who discloses current domestic violence. One commonly used risk assessment checklist can be found in Appendix B. Risk assessments should ideally be carried out by someone who has been appropriately trained in their use. Remember that risk levels can change – sometimes quite rapidly – and that they are never foolproof.

If it appears that the patient is in *immediate danger* then it might be necessary to call the police and/or other emergency services. If a patient is frightened to return home, referral to a refuge service (either locally or out of the area in order to increase the patient's safety) might be the best option.

If the danger seems *less immediate*, support staff working for specialist domestic abuse services can help the patient develop a safety plan (see next section).

When a patient *appears to reject help* (see Box 9.2), it is harder to deal with; but it is important to make it clear that help is available when she is ready for it and that she can come back to you at any time. It might be worth making a follow-up appointment to talk again, or talking to a specialist agency for your own support and to get some other ideas.

> Box 9.2 **Case study: Dawn O'Connor**
>
> Whenever Dawn came to the GP surgery she was accompanied by her husband, Tony. Tony always seemed very solicitous, even standing outside when she went to the toilet. Once when she went to collect her prescription from the on-site pharmacy, she was heard having to ask him for money to pay for it.
>
> Dawn had a couple of miscarriages, and the nurse asked Tony to wait outside while she undertook a full internal examination and smear. She took the opportunity to ask Dawn whether she was experiencing any abuse. Dawn told her that Tony was 'sometimes a bit overprotective' and didn't like her seeing her family, but that he hadn't hurt her at all. On further questioning, she admitted that he had pushed her once or twice, and that she was sometimes afraid of him. The nurse offered her a leaflet but Dawn refused to take it, and seemed rather scared. The nurse had concerns, but did not know what else to do and felt she could do nothing more.
>
> Two months later, Dawn was found strangled in her own home. Tony pleaded guilty to manslaughter on the grounds of 'provocation'.

When *risk levels seem high*, referral to an MARAC might also be considered.

The Royal College of General Practitioners (RCGP), in association with Coordinated Action Against Domestic Abuse (CAADA) and Identification and Referral to Improve Safety (IRIS), has produced guidance to help GPs respond effectively to patients experiencing domestic violence and abuse (DVA); see http://www.rcgp.org.uk/clinical-and-research/clinical-resources/domestic-violence.aspx (last accessed 12 February 2014).

Overview of specialist violence support services

How to find an appropriate support service

The RCGP guidance for general practices recommends that a designated person in each practice should investigate what domestic violence services are available locally and engage with them to develop an effective working partnership. This advice is relevant to all health care settings. Developing clear referrals and pathways and ensuring that everyone (including reception staff) is aware of these is an important first step in providing support.

Most specialist domestic violence services are run by the voluntary sector. Women's Aid coordinates an England-wide network of more than 300 organisations, providing around 500 local support services (see Box 9.3), and there are similar networks in Wales, Scotland and Northern Ireland. These include outreach, advocacy, floating support, sexual abuse support services, resettlement services, refuge accommodation and support and services for children affected by domestic abuse.

Unfortunately, service provision is not available equally throughout the country, and, due to funding cuts, many existing services are under threat. One in four local authorities has no specialised domestic violence support services, and only one in ten local authority areas has a specialised service for women from black and minority ethnic (BME) communities. If you are unable to find a local service, survivors should be referred to the 24-hour Freephone National Domestic Violence Helpline (see Box 9.4).

Box 9.4 **Case study: Shabnam Patel**

Shabnam comes to see you in great distress. She has several bruises on her arms and legs, and says her husband grabbed her and tried to throw her downstairs yesterday and has threatened to kill her. You give her contact numbers for the local refuge organisation and for the National Helpline and say she can come back and talk to you, or to the practice nurse, at any time. You also offer a quiet office where she can use the phone and make the calls in privacy.

A few weeks later she comes back to the surgery. She seems much happier and says she has found as place in a specialist refuge for South Asian women. They are providing ongoing support for her and her daughter.

What kinds of specialist support service are available?

Refuge-based services

These provide a package of temporary accommodation, support, information and advocacy for women who have experienced domestic violence and for their children. The majority of refuges are provided within the voluntary sector, either by independent women-run organisations or by larger organisations such as housing associations.

Outreach, floating support and other non-refuge-based services

These provide a wide range of advocacy and support, including:

- Resettlement services – enabling women and their children to make new lives in the community after leaving refuge.
- Drop-in centres.
- Survivors' support groups.
- Telephone helplines.

- Counselling services for those who have experienced domestic and sexual violence.
- Specialist court advocacy services.
- Independent Domestic violence Advisors (IDVAs).
- Independent Sexual Violence Advisors (ISVAs).
- Floating support services, providing advocacy and support to families.

Why women-only services?

Some non-refuge-based services provide support for both female and male victims of domestic violence – ideally at separate times. Some of them also provide specialist support services for children and young people who have experienced domestic abuse, either from adults in their families (directly or indirectly) or within their own relationships. Most services, however – particularly refuge provision and other accommodation-based services – are for women and their children only.

DVA is disproportionately experienced by women, most of whom prefer (or need) to access support services run by female staff. Women-only services provide physical and emotional safety and security for those who have experienced abuse, as well as offering empathy, solidarity and understanding. Women-only services can often reach women who would not use mainstream services. Those from BME communities might also prefer BME-specific services, where these are available.

MARACs, IDVAs and SDVCs

Multi-Agency Risk Assessment Conferences (MARACs)

MARACs aim to coordinate action in order to increase the safety of high-risk victims of domestic violence by holding regular meetings of representatives of all relevant agencies, such as the police, local authority housing services, domestic and sexual violence specialist support services and so on. Health care professionals – including those from mental health and drug and alcohol services – may also be invited. The objective is to prevent further abuse by better sharing of information and providing and coordinating a multi-agency response. This should be seen as a means to an end – i.e. providing effective, coordinated support services – rather than the end in itself.

Research to date suggests that the introduction of MARACs has been effective in reducing revictimisation of survivors and enhancing the safety of staff working with violent perpetrators, as well as in information sharing. A cost–benefit analysis has further suggested that if MARACs were established throughout the country, they would save £740 million of public money annually due to their effectiveness in preventing repeat incidents, as there are already direct costs to agencies in contact with high-risk victims such as the police, health, housing and children's services (approximately £6 saved for every £1 invested) (CAADA, 2012a, 2012b). However, there have been some reservations over the use of MARACs, from both practitioners and victims.

There may be times when you might consider referring a patient to your local MARAC. Referrals should follow your local protocols, which will identify the patient's level of risk ('threshold') .

Professional judgment should be taken very seriously, however, and an individual might be referred even when they do not appear to meet the formal criteria for 'high risk'.

Independent Domestic Violence Advisors (IDVAs)

IDVAs are primarily aimed at providing support and information to high-risk victims and are usually linked to criminal justice interventions and to MARACs. They therefore normally work with their clients from the point of crisis in the short- and medium-term, in order to help them towards long-term safety. Some IDVAs are also based within health services or within specialist domestic violence organisations, and they may support a wider range of victims (see Box 9.5).

Box 9.5 **Case study: Beverley Cohen**

Beverley turns up in A&E with a bad scald on her arm, which occurred 3 days ago. At first she says it was an accident, but eventually she reluctantly discloses that her husband, Bill, poured boiling water over her arm because he was angry that she was talking on the phone to her mother when he came home from work, rather than being ready with a cup of tea for him. She insists this is the first time he has done something like this and that he was very repentant. You give her a contact card and suggest that she talk to the IDVA based in the hospital to discuss options 'just in case it happens again; or maybe a friend of yours might need the number and advice'.

IDVAs have a specific remit to represent victims at MARACs and help implement the actions of the MARAC. They also assess levels of risk, discuss the range of suitable options, help survivors develop safety plans and support them through the criminal and civil courts. Their involvement is therefore usually short-term and at the point of crisis. However, they may also refer survivors to other support services that are available for a longer period.

Specialist Domestic Violence Courts (SDVCs)

These were set up to make it easier for victims to give evidence against their abusers. SDVC magistrates, legal advisors and court staff are specially trained in domestic violence, and there are special in-court arrangements for victims, such as safe waiting areas and enhanced victim/witness services.

Table 9.1 sets out some of the main sources of practical help that a survivor might need. Clearly, not everyone will choose to take up the services offered, or not at this point. Except where children or vulnerable adults are at risk of serious harm, this choice should be left to the person concerned.

Those disclosing abuse could also be referred to the Women's Aid Survivor's Handbook, which is available in different languages and has an audio version: http://www.womensaid.org.uk/domestic-violence-survivors-handbook.asp?section=0001000100080001&sectionTitle=The+Survivor%27s+Handbook (last accessed 12 February 2014).

Table 9.1 Summary of specialist and nonspecialist services.

	Current or ongoing abuse	Historic abuse
Refuge service	✓	–
Outreach support	✓	✓
IDVA/advocacy	✓	✓
Other specialist domestic violence service	✓	✓
Housing /homeless department	✓	-
Police/criminal justice system	✓	✓
MARAC	✓	-
Legal advice	✓	✓
Counselling or other mental health support	✓	✓
Social care children and young people services	✓	✓
Vulnerable adults teams	✓	✓
Other, e.g. welfare benefits advice, substance use service, immigration advice, etc.	✓	✓

Domestic homicide reviews

DVA often results in serious injury, and in some cases in death by suicide or murder. On average, two women a week are killed by a current or former male partner (Coleman *et al.*, 2010, 2011). The incident that results in the death of the victim is very rarely the first violent attack: there is likely to have been a previous ongoing pattern of physical and/or psychological abuse, and a number of agencies (e.g. police, health professionals) might have been aware of this through their contacts with the victim.

In 2011, Section 9 of the Domestic Violence, Crime and Victims Act 2004 was implemented, introducing a legal requirement for a domestic homicide review to be carried out following a domestic violence-related homicide. The purpose is to review any interventions or support provided by agencies involved with the victim before her death in order to assess the effectiveness or otherwise of their procedures. Reviews are carried out by community safety partnerships and are not intended to establish how the victim died or who is to blame (which is a matter for coroners and criminal courts) but to provide an opportunity to learn from mistakes made, improve individual and collective responses and prevent future tragedies. The ultimate aim is to improve practice, and hence avoid future incidents of domestic homicide.

The Home Office has issued Multi-Agency Statutory Guidance for the Conduct of Domestic Homicide Reviews, outlining when and how a review should be carried out. This is available at http://www.homeoffice.gov.uk/publications/crime/DHR-guidance (last accessed 12 February 2014).

Advocacy After Fatal Domestic Abuse (www.aafda.org.uk, last accessed 12 February 2014) is a charity that helps families affected by domestic homicide. It can support families in contributing to a review, where required.

Further reading

CAADA (2010) *Saving Lives, Saving Money: MARACs and High Risk Domestic Abuse*, http://www.caada.org.uk/research/research.html (last accessed 12 February 2014).

CAADA (2012a) A place of greater safety, http://www.caada.org.uk/policy/A_Place_of_greater_safety.pdf (last accessed 12 February 2014).

CAADA (2012b) Saving lives, saving money: MARACs and high risk domestic abuse, http://www.caada.org.uk/policy/Saving_lives_saving_money_FINAL_REFERENCED_VERSION.pdf (last accessed 12 February 2014).

Coleman, K., Eder, S. & Smith, K. (2011) Homicide, in Smith, K., Coleman, K., Eder, S. & Hall, P. (eds) Home Office Statistical Bulletin 01/11: Homicides, Firearm Offences and Intimate Violence 2009/10. *Supplementary Volume 2 to Crime in England and Wales 2009/10*. Home Office, London, http://rds.homeoffice.gov.uk/rds/pdfs11/hosb0111.pdf (last accessed 12 February 2014).

Coleman, K. & Osborne, S. (2010) Homicide. In: Smith, K., Coleman, K., Eder, S. & Hall, P. (eds) *Homicides, Firearm Offences and Intimate Violence 2008–9. Supplementary Volume 2 to Crime in England and Wales 2008/9*. Home Office, London.

Coy, M., Kelly, L. & Foord, J. (2009) *Map of Gaps 2: The Postcode Lottery of Violence Against Women Support Services in Britain*. EVAW in partnership with Equality and Human Rights Commission, London.

Douglas, N., Lilley, S.J., Kooper, L. & Diamond, A. (2004) *Safety and Justice: Sharing Personal Information in the Context of Domestic Violence – An Overview*. Home Office Development and Practice Report 30, London.

Farthing, R. (2012) Multi-agency risk assessment conferences: a review in Birmingham. *Safe*, **41**, 21–24.

Imkaan (2008) *A matter of Life and Death: The Loss of Specialist Services for BAMER Women and Children Experiencing Domestic Abuse*. Imkaan, London.

Robinson, A. (2006) Reducing repeat victimisation among high-risk victims of DV: the benefits of a co-ordinated community response in Cardiff, Wales. *Violence Against Women*, **12**(8), 761–788.

Robinson, A. (2009) *Independent Domestic Violence Advisors: A Process Evaluation*. University of Cardiff, Cardiff; funded by Home Office, http://www.cardiff.ac.uk/socsi/research/researchprojects/violenceadvisors.html (last accessed 12 February 2014).

Towers, J. & Walby, S. (2012) *Measuring the Impact of Cuts in Public Expenditure on the Provision of Services to Prevent Violence against Women and Girls*. Trust for London and Northern Rock Foundation, London, http://www.trustforlondon.org.uk/VAWG%20Full%20report.pdf (last accessed 12 February 2014).

Women's Resource Centre (2007) *Why Women-Only? The Value and Benefits of By Women, For Women Services*. Women's Resource Centre, London.

CHAPTER 10

Perpetrators

Colin Fitzgerald and Jo Todd

Respect, UK

Why should I be concerned about this issue?

Most perpetrators of domestic violence will not come into contact with the criminal justice system – but many seek help for their behaviour.

In a small-scale study, researchers found that most men who sought help for their violent or abusive behaviour initially went to their GP but presented with a secondary concern such as depression or anxiety. Skilful practitioners may be able to point their patients to relevant sources for help rather than 'mislabelling' or 'medicalising' the actual underlying problem.

This chapter concentrates largely on male perpetrators of domestic violence as this is the most common and most researched group. Although there is thought to be great overlap and common traits between them, we cannot assume that perpetrators of domestic and of sexual violence share the same characteristics, nor that male and female perpetrators are similar. Nevertheless, simple practical skills should help health professionals deal with relevant issues for all these groups.

Look and listen during presentation

Some perpetrators will recognise their violent and abusive behaviour and ask for help – though usually they will have been motivated by a possible consequence. For example, their partner

may have threatened to leave if they don't seek help, the worst incident of violence and abuse may recently have taken place or there may be impending criminal justice proceedings.

Very few perpetrators of domestic violence will state clearly that they are a perpetrator, even when help-seeking (see Box 10.1).

Box 10.1 **Perpetrator presentation**

Ways in which perpetrators of abuse and violence might present themselves

- They are having problems in their relationship or at home.
- They have a problem with their anger.
- They are depressed.
- They perpetrate violence, but present themselves as the victim or suggest that the violence is mutual.[1]
- Most will not mention their abuse at all. Instead they will present with a 'mitigating' factor such as depression, anxiety or alcohol/substance misuse.

You may discover a patient is a perpetrator through another route

- Through an information sharing protocol or process such as a MARAC (Multi-Agency Risk Assessment Conference) or Child Protection.
- Because their partner has presented as a victim.

You may suspect someone is a perpetrator through their behaviour

- Someone who *insists* on accompanying their partner to an appointment.
- And then *talks for* them.
- Or where their *partner or children appear afraid* of them.

[1]Although most perpetrators are men abusing female partners, there are also female perpetrators who abuse male partners and perpetrators in same-sex relationships. Male victims can contact the Men's Advice Line, free, on 0808 801 0327 or at www.mensadviceline.org.uk for support and practical advice.

Ask questions

If you are presented with 'mitigating factors', such as drinking, stress or depression, it may be useful to ask:

- 'How is this [drinking/stress at work/depression/anger] affecting how you are with your family?'
- 'When you feel like that, how do you behave?'
- 'Do you find yourself shouting or smashing things?'

ABC of Domestic and Sexual Violence, First Edition.
Edited by Susan Bewley and Jan Welch.
© 2014 John Wiley & Sons, Ltd. Published 2014 by John Wiley & Sons, Ltd.

- 'Do you ever feel aggressive or violent towards a particular person?'
- 'It sounds like you want to make some changes, for your own benefit and for the sake of your [partner/child/parent]. What choices do you have? What can you do about it? What help would assist you to make these changes?'

If domestic abuse has been explicitly stated as an issue, it may be useful to ask:

- 'It sounds as though your behaviour can be frightening; does your partner say she is frightened of you?'
- 'How are the children affected?'
- 'Have the police ever been called to the house because of your behaviour?'
- 'What worries you most about your behaviour?'
- 'Who else might be frightened of you?'

Think about risk

Certain factors and/or combinations of factors can indicate the likelihood of serious harm or homicide towards a partner, ex-partner or children:

- High levels of coercive control.
- Grabbing by the throat or strangulation.
- The victim indicating they are in fear for their life.
- Threats to kill or the use of weapons.
- Stalking, harassment, high levels of jealousy.
- Pregnancy.
- Substance/alcohol misuse.
- Escalation of levels of violence and increase in frequency.
- Continuation despite the intervention of services.

Direct questions relating to heightened risk factors may sometimes be appropriate:

- 'Do you feel unhappy about your partner seeing friends or family; do you ever try to stop her?'
- 'Have you assaulted your partner in front of the children?'
- 'Have you ever assaulted or threatened your partner with a knife or other weapon?'
- 'Did your behaviour change/has your behaviour changed towards your partner during pregnancy?'
- 'What has been the worst occasion of violence?'
- 'Have you ever grabbed your partner by the throat?'
- 'Do you feel that your behaviour has got worse?'

Multi-agency risk assessment conferences (MARACs) are meetings at which information about high-risk domestic abuse victims (those at risk of murder or serious harm) is shared between local agencies (see Chapter 9). You should be aware of your local MARAC and when and how to refer someone; see www.caada.org.uk for further information. By bringing all agencies together at a MARAC, a risk-focused, coordinated safety plan can be drawn up to support the victim.

Respond and refer

Before offering an intervention, ask yourself, 'Does the intervention I'm offering increase the safety of the victim and their children or have I just made it easier for the abuser to abuse?' In other words, be careful to *do no further harm*.

To this end, you should look to work with services that are focused on victim and child safety and that support perpetrators of violence in becoming accountable for their behaviour. The dos and don'ts listed in Box 10.2 may help guide your actions and responses.

Box 10.2 **Some practical dos and don'ts regarding perpetrators**

Do

- Remember that an abuser is always 100% responsible for his actions.
- Be aware of barriers to his seeking help – such as shame, guilt and self-justifying anger.
- Give clear messages that abusive behaviour is not acceptable: it is harmful to his partner and children and may be criminal.
- Motivate him to change; reassure him that there is help available.
- Encourage him to call the Respect phoneline (freephone 0808 802 4040) or visit the Web site (www.respectphoneline.org.uk) for support, or call yourself for professional advice.
- Refer him to a local domestic violence prevention programme (DVPP) that has Respect membership (the Respect phoneline has details).

Don't

- Refer him to anger management – most domestic violence perpetrators manage their anger well. What they need support with is understanding why they use violence and abuse within the context of their relationship. Additionally, without the advent of linked partner support for the victim, this is likely to be unsafe as an intervention.
- Refer him for couple counselling. This locates the abuse with the couple rather than 100% with the abuser. The victim is unlikely to be able to talk freely for fear of possible consequences and retribution and so her safety will be further diminished.

Confidentiality and the safety of others

There is a professional duty to maintain confidentiality of information obtained within the intimate and private doctor–patient relationship, but this is not an absolute duty if there are serious risks to other individuals (see General Medical Council guidance in the Further Reading). It is not easy to assess the risk your patient poses to others, or how far your responsibilities to prevent future harm go. How serious is the threat a patient makes when he says something like, 'Sometimes I feel like strangling her,' or admits following his ex-partner around and threatening her in public? You must take concerns about others' safety seriously and be able to justify your actions. If you are considering disclosing information, make a reflective judgement, as information sharing may be life-saving but breaching confidentiality may be dangerous to others and to yourself. There are many sources of help, but no simple formulaic response, as each case is different and

Table 10.1 Personal safety, conflict and security at work. Adapted from Australian Federation of Medical Women, http://afmw.org.au (last accessed 12 February 2014).

Professional consultation skills	• Take your fears seriously. • Be aware of signs of agitation. • Learn about conflict resolution and de-escalation tactics. • Use your professional skills: calm voice, polite language, non-intimidating body language. • Avoid escalation, threatening behaviour and expression of anger. • Make an excuse to get 'time out' or a break in the consultation. • Offer to get help, third parties or more senior people involved. • If endangered, call for help and get out.
Workplace responsibility	**Risk assessment and controls** • Consult with security expert. • Assess whether measures can be taken to increase workplace security. **Incident logging and review** • Record as soon as possible. • Ensure appropriate debriefing for all staff if a safety issue occurs. **Complaints procedure** • Use to defuse tension. • Make visible and ensure it is acted upon. **Policy on violence** • Make personal safety and security a regular agenda item for staff meetings. • Implement human resources policies on lone workers, bullying, harassment and violence at work.
Consider exposures to risk	These include: • After-hours consulting with little or no support staff. • Lone home visits. • Unstable drug seekers demanding prescriptions. • Consultation with aggressive or unstable patients. • Stalking (e.g. nuisance phone calls, text messages, being followed).
Ways to mitigate the risks to your personal safety	**Are you safe at work, and getting to and from work?** • Examine room layouts, doors and escape routes. • Secure items that might be used as weapons (e.g. computer monitor, printer, scissors, letter openers). • Only consult when another staff member is nearby or in earshot. • Ensure adequate lighting when walking to your transport. • Park closer to the building at the end of the day. **Can you call for help?** • Have a laminated list of emergency numbers near office phones. • Keep a phone charger at work, at home and in the car. • Ensure all practice phones and staff mobiles are programmed with emergency numbers on speed dial. • Install alarm buttons under the consultation desk and have them monitored by reception staff and security via on-line phone surveillance. • Wear a duress alarm when you are alone and in situations where you believe your personal safety is at risk. **Does someone know where you are or when to help you?** • Have protocols and action plans on how to manage a duress call from reception or a consulting room. • Provide regular staff training/safety drills to ensure a quick, automatic response. • Link a speaker phone to a one-dial automated process so that reception staff can hear what is going on in the consultation room. • Advise someone of your anticipated time of return if you attend patients out of hours. • Use a deputising service out of hours or ensure a support person attends with you. Have an agreed plan in the event of a threat to your safety. **Anticipate and plan** • If you are aware of a potentially difficult encounter, agree on a time when a staff member is to knock and enter to check on you. • Seek additional professional support if a patient threatens suicide. • Be mindful of after-hours calls for pain relief without appropriate assessment. **Keep appropriate professional boundaries** • Listen carefully and take patients' concerns seriously. • 'Friendly' is not the same as 'a friend'. • Do not use a personal mobile to call patients. • If you give patients and carers your professional email address, use a separate one not linked to any social media you use (e.g. Facebook). • Programme a 'caller number display' on your mobile and landline; use an answerphone to screen calls. • Consider having your home phone number ex-directory and use a professional rather than a home address for the General Medical Council etc. • Document all text/phone calls in the patient record.

nuanced. You should review General Medical Council guidance, local safeguarding and information-sharing policies and talk things through with senior colleagues and your medical defence organisation.

Patients who frighten you

It is important for health professionals to stay safe themselves. There are patients who can intimidate, threaten and frighten. We understand that sometimes patients behave bizarrely because they are very ill, delirious or hallucinating, psychotic or brain-damaged, or because they themselves are frightened. Sometimes aggression is deliberate – the patient may want something specific and that is how they deal with everyone. While, inevitably, patients and carers can be ill, confused, frightened or upset and this can cause them to 'act out', abusive, aggressive and violent behaviour should not be tolerated. It is totally unacceptable that any member of a health care team should be subject to verbal threats or physical violence. There are techniques and courses that can help develop skills for conflict reduction and resolution. See Table 10.1 for ideas regarding safety, conflict and security at work.

Further reading

Hester, M. & Westmarland, N. (2006) Domestic violence perpetrators. *Criminal Justice Matters*, **66**(1), 34–35.

General Medical Council (no date) Duties of a doctor, http://www .gmc-uk.org/guidance/good_medical_practice/duties_of_a_doctor.asp (last accessed 12 February 2014).

Westmarland, N., Kelly, L. & Chalder-Mills, J. (2010) Domestic violence perpetrator programmes: what counts as success?, http://www.respect.uk.net/ data/files/respect_research_briefing_note_1_what_counts_as_success.pdf (last accessed 12 February 2014).

CHAPTER 11

General Practice

Emmeline Brew-Graves

General Practice, Southway Surgery, UK

OVERVIEW
- Domestic violence and abuse are common and hidden
- The majority of 'victims' are female
- The majority of general practice consultations are with women, making this an ideal location for detection and intervention

Common presentations in general practice

Apart from the obvious case of attendance with a clear history or injury, domestic violence should be considered in other scenarios, such as those listed in Box 11.1. Also consider routinely enquiring about domestic abuse at antenatal appointments, postnatal checks, pill checks, cervical screening or when a sexually transmitted infection (STI) screen or emergency contraception is requested.

Box 11.1 **'Red flags' for abuse and violence presenting in a general practice consultation**

- The frequent attender at the surgery/the frequent attender elsewhere – remember emergency departments (A&E) and out of hours contact letters/slips. The frequent attender often presents with:
  - Vague symptoms.
  - Depression, anxiety, self-harm or psychosomatic symptoms.
- Patients who frequently attend as an 'emergency' but do not attend scheduled appointments.
- Frequently missed appointments.
- Injuries inconsistent with the explanation given.
- Injuries that are hidden (e.g. to the breast or abdomen) or minimised.
- The subdued or silent patient always accompanied by a family member who talks on the patient's behalf without reference to them.

Asking the question

Enquire directly but sensitively about domestic abuse. This must be in a safe place, with no other family members, including children (except the very young), present. If an interpreter is needed, do not use a family member.

Use the HARK questions (see Chapter 7, Box 7.7) and make a note of the date and time in the patient records.

Managing a disclosure of domestic violence

There are four main factors:

- Focus on the here and now.
- Remain calm.
- Listen carefully.
- Record what you are told using the patient's own words.

Assess the situation

Ask yourself:

- Is there an immediate and significant risk?
- Has a crime been committed?
- Are the emergency services (ambulance or police) required?
- Are the safety and well being of your patient in jeopardy?
- Are the safety and well being of any children in jeopardy?
- Is your role today to provide support and advice?

Ask your patient:

- 'Are you safe to go home?'
- 'Are either you or the children in danger?'
- 'Has violence become more frequent or severe recently?'
- 'Are there any weapons in the home? For example, a bread knife or a hammer?'
- 'Have there been threats to kill [you/your children/your pets]?'

ABC of Domestic and Sexual Violence, First Edition.
Edited by Susan Bewley and Jan Welch.
© 2014 John Wiley & Sons, Ltd. Published 2014 by John Wiley & Sons, Ltd.

Box 11.2 provides some indications of high-risk cases.

> Box 11.2 **High-risk cases**
>
> Women are at greatest risk:
>
> - At the point of separation and afterwards.
> - If there is sexual violence, strangulation, threats to kill or use of weapons.
> - After separation; 76% of domestic violence homicides occur following separation.
>
> Children are at greater risk:
>
> - If they are under the age of 7 years.
> - If their mother is pregnant.
> - If either the mother or the child has special needs.

Safeguarding children and vulnerable adults

Inform your patient that you are required to share certain information, explaining what will be shared and why. Keep your statements relatively simple: 'I am worried about you', 'I am worried about your child', 'Even if he is sorry, this can happen again and again and get more serious'.

Domestic violence is a child protection issue

You can seek advice (without necessarily disclosing the identity of the individual) from an experienced colleague, local safeguarding/domestic violence lead or medical defence organisation. If a rape is alleged, consider seeking advice from your local sexual assault referral centre (SARC).

Articulating your concerns to another professional often crystallises a way forward.

Examine the patient if physical violence is disclosed

Use diagrams to document any injuries. If police involvement is rejected, advise the patient to photograph injuries or consider photographing the injuries at the practice or the local hospital medical photography department.

Management plan

- Do not assume that domestic violence spells the end of the relationship.
- Treat any injuries that can be managed in primary care.
- Discuss a management plan and seek consent for appropriate information sharing.
- Arrange referrals: hospital referrals, safeguarding referrals and referral to a local domestic violence organisation. Local domestic violence agencies have independent domestic violence advisors (IDVAs) who can support the patient via advocacy; they can also broker access to housing, and provide criminal justice and social care support.

- If you are familiar with the CAADA-DASH Questionnaire (Coordinated Action Against Domestic Abuse & Domestic Abuse, Stalking and 'Honour'-Based Violence), it may be appropriate to complete it at this encounter or to consider arranging another appointment to complete it (see Appendix B).
- Discuss safety planning and safety numbers.
- Make sure the patient leaves with the 24 hour National Domestic Violence Helpline number (0808 2000 247) and the numbers of any local domestic violence organisations.
- Consider a referral to the local multi-agency risk assessment conference (MARAC; see Box 11.3 and Chapter 9).

> Box 11.3 **The Multi-Agency Risk Assessment Conference (MARAC)**
>
> - MARACs are multidisciplinary meetings at which information about high-risk domestic abuse victims (those at risk of murder or serious harm) is shared between local agencies.
> - The participating agencies will usually represent health, social care, the police and local domestic violence voluntary agencies.
> - By bringing all agencies together at a MARAC, a risk-focused, coordinated safety plan can be drawn up to support the victim.
> - Over 260 MARACs currently operate across England, Wales and Northern Ireland, managing over 57 000 cases a year.
> - Your local MARAC team can be found at http://www.caada.org.uk/marac/findamarac.html (last accessed 12 February 2014).
> - MARAC meetings are convened regularly; some meetings are monthly, some twice a month.
> - The aim is to:
>   - Share information in order to increase the safety, health and well being of victims/survivors: adults and their children.
>   - Determine whether the alleged perpetrator poses a significant risk to any particular individual or to the general community.
>   - Jointly construct and implement a risk-management plan that provides professional support to all those at risk and reduces the risk of harm.
>   - Reduce repeat victimisation.
>   - Improve agency accountability.
>   - Improve support for staff involved in high-risk domestic abuse cases.

After the consultation

- Consider proactive communication with local GP out of hours services.
- Make use of any sources of advice.
- If the patient does not give her consent for referrals, confidentiality may be broken when safeguarding vulnerable individuals.
- There must be clear justification where action is taken without consent (e.g. lack of capacity, best interests, other legal reasons, public interest justification).
- Referrals to social and health care services for concerns about child abuse need to be made in writing within 48 hours of the decision to refer.

- Work at maintaining a safe, confidential, trusting doctor–patient relationship even in the face of return to an abuser, as it may take time to build up confidence.

Practice response

- Make sure there are domestic violence awareness posters/leaflets in the waiting room – this may encourage disclosure.
- Does the practice have a practice safeguarding (including domestic violence) champion? If not, why not?
- Locum pack: make sure there is a useful telephone number for the lone locum in a single-handed practice to call for advice.
- The Royal College of General Practitioners (RCGP) has produced a handy flowchart (see Chapters 3 and 7).
- All members of the primary health care team should regularly attend safeguarding children, safeguarding vulnerable adults and domestic violence training.

Case studies are provided in Boxes 11.4 and 11.5.

Box 11.4 **Case study**

Mirabelle Ngozi is a 36-year-old immigrant from Africa who is in the UK on a spousal visa. She has no children. Her husband has a 3-year-old son by a previous partner who comes to visit but does not stay with them. She works as a chambermaid in a hotel. Her husband controls her bank account as he has told her they need to save to self-fund IVF treatment. She has no key to their home so has to wait outside, in all weathers, until her husband comes home from work.

She comes to the surgery because last night her husband hit her for not being outside when he got home. He accused her of being unfaithful. She has no documented past medical history. She has no family in the UK. Everyone she knows in the UK she has met through her husband. This is the first time she has attended the surgery unaccompanied by her husband.

Here and now

She has disclosed domestic abuse. On being asked the HARK questions, she admits to submitting to sexual assault as she is desperate to get pregnant. Her husband frequently humiliates her in private and in public and mocks her because she has not become pregnant; he tells her it is her fault. As he has a son already, he knows it is not his fault.

- Her narrative, the date and time of the consultation should be documented.
- On assessment, she does not feel she is in immediate danger. She does not think there are any weapons in the house.
- As her stepson does not live or stay with them, he is in no immediate danger. However, a safeguarding referral ought to be considered and discussed.
- The situation is discussed with a senior colleague, who suggests a local advocacy organisation that specializes in immigration issues.
- She is examined. Her injuries are minor and need no active treatment. They are documented on body diagrams. Her mobile phone has a camera, so she is happy to photograph the injuries with a ruler in view.

- She does not want to end the relationship as she is in the process of organising IVF and feels this may be her only chance to have her own child.

Management plan

- *Safety planning*: As she has no trusted friend to go to if she needs a place of safety, Mirabelle is given the number for the National Domestic Violence Helpline, which she stores in her mobile phone under the name 'Jane Doe'. She agrees to retrieve her passport and keep it at work with her line manager. She also agrees to be referred to the local advocacy service. A follow-up appointment is scheduled for 1 month's time at the GP practice.
- *After the consultation*: The GP performs a structured Personal Reflection on Mirabelle's management. He discusses his concerns with the practice team at the clinical meeting and the decision is taken that a 'safeguarding children' referral ought to be made. The local safeguarding lead suggests that a referral be made to the local borough children's services.

Box 11.5 **Case study 2**

Jack and Jill Taylor are a white British couple with no children who have been together for 3 years. One day they have a blazing row. Even though there is no physical violence, Jill is very frightened. They break up and Jill moves out to stay with a friend. After a month of communicating by telephone they agree to meet up in a restaurant on a Saturday. They have a pleasant evening and Jack offers to take Jill back to where she is staying. On leaving the restaurant, Jill realises that Jack is driving in the wrong direction, so she suggests that she drives. Jack stops the car in a wooded area. He gets out of the driver's side of the car. As Jill is getting out of the passenger side, Jack pushes her back into the seat, pulls down her shorts and underwear and has vaginal sex with her without a condom. Jill tries to push him off but is not able to. When it is over, he drives off and leaves her. She walks first in high heels then barefoot to the nearest bus stop. She has abrasions to her feet. Jill presents to her GP first thing on Monday morning (2 days after the incident) as an emergency walk-in patient (5 minute slots) to request emergency contraception. She looks subdued. How would you proceed?

Possible course of action

Ask the question: '*Jill, I hope you do not mind me asking, but you look so sad. How are things at home?*' Write down what she says. Ensure the entry has the date and time.

Managing a disclosure of domestic violence starts with the here and now (assessing the situation):

- Jill is staying with a friend, so she is safe.
- A crime has been committed (rape/nonconsensual sexual intercourse).
- What is the role of the health care professional today? (If unsure, seek advice from an experienced colleague, local domestic violence or adult safeguarding lead or the local SARC.)
- Assess Jill's need for emergency contraception and provide it.

- Examine her for injuries and document them carefully.
- Make referrals, e.g. to a sexual health clinic (if she requires this or requests an intrauterine contraceptive device and it is not provided at the practice), the local SARC and/or the police.
- Issue a medical certificate (Med3) if her injuries are severe enough to warrant time off work.

Management plan

- Discuss your management plan and options with Jill and seek her consent for appropriate information sharing.
- Arrange referrals.
- Arrange a follow-up appointment to review her for emergency contraception failure and for ongoing support needs, e.g. referral for counselling and STI screening.
- Document the consultation fully and contemporaneously.

Further reading

The Havens (2010) Where Is Your Line?, http://www.youtube.com/watch?v=j3TT0TfQHKM (last accessed 12 February 2014).

Royal College of General Practitioners (no date) Domestic violence, http://www.rcgp.org.uk/policy/rcgp-policy-areas/domestic-violence.aspx (last accessed 12 February 2014).

Sohal, H., Eldridge, S. & Feder, G. (2007) The sensitivity and specificity of four questions (HARK) to identify intimate partner violence: a diagnostic accuracy study in general practice. *BMC Family Practice*, **8**, 49.

CHAPTER 12

Emergency Medicine and Surgical Specialities

Lindsey Stevens

Department of Emergency Medicine, Epsom and St Helier University NHS Trust, UK

OVERVIEW

- 1–4% patients attending emergency departments in the UK 'have come that day as a direct result of domestic violence; a quarter have experienced domestic violence in their lifetime'
- One in six rape victims present first to an emergency department
- Patients do not present just with injuries but also with overdoses, psychiatric illnesses, substance abuse, somatisation and requests for postcoital contraception. Child abuse is closely related to abuse of the mother
- Useful indicators include delay in presentation, injuries inconsistent with story, frequent attendance and failure to wait to be seen
- Interview patients alone and ask directly and nonjudgmentally about abuse. If the patient is returning to the abuser, discuss an 'exit plan' and risk assessment. Refer high-risk patients to the local multiagency risk assessment conference (MARAC)
- Forensic evidence is vital. Involve the forensic medical examiner or sexual assault referral centre (SARC) at the earliest opportunity and keep meticulous clinical notes. Advise patients on the preservation of evidence and collect early evidence when necessary
- Offer patients attending after sexual violence viral and bacterial infection prophylaxis as appropriate and arrange follow up in the SARC or genitourinary medicine clinic
- Offer all patients experiencing violence psychosocial support during their attendance and after discharge. Staff members seeing such patients should also be offered debriefing and counselling

Emergency medicine and surgical specialties

Around 15 million people every year use UK emergency departments as their first point of contact with health services. This is particularly true of vulnerable patients whose social situations and psychological states militate against using planned care. Studies in the UK put the incidence of domestic violence presenting to general emergency departments at 1.2–4.2%. One in six rape cases present initially to emergency departments. Staff members therefore have a unique opportunity to identify and support patients who are suffering the results of domestic and sexual violence and to provide crisis intervention when invited. Sadly, such abuse often goes unsuspected; even where it is suspected, lack of confidence, protocols and time may mean that staff members sidestep the issue. Treating a patient with domestic or sexual violence is distressing for clinicians, particularly those with personal experience of abuse; staff members should be supported within the team and by staff counsellors.

When to suspect domestic and sexual violence in the emergency department

The first pitfall is the assumption that domestic and sexual violence always present as trauma (Box 12.1). In fact, they present in a wide variety of ways, and the incidence and prevalence are far higher than is evident if only injury is considered.

Box 12.1 **Characteristic injuries**

Pointers: multiple, symmetrical distribution to areas that are normally covered and spiral or healing fractures

- Head/facial injury, perforated eardrums, detached retina.
- Upper-limb injury.
- Neck/back injury.
- Burns/scalds/bruises/bites/bizarre injuries.
- Rape, genital injury, vaginal bleeding, postcoital contraception.
- Breast injury.
- Abdominal injury when pregnant, abruption.

Domestic and sexual violence, whether experienced as a child or an adult, are common underlying factors in 'heartsink' patients. Some patients turn to alcohol and drug abuse to cope with the violence, some somatise their distress and some turn to the emergency department again and again. Some patients present to the surgical specialties in the out-patient clinic (Box 12.2).

ABC of Domestic and Sexual Violence, First Edition.
Edited by Susan Bewley and Jan Welch.
© 2014 John Wiley & Sons, Ltd. Published 2014 by John Wiley & Sons, Ltd.

Box 12.2 **Nontrauma presentations to surgical specialities**

- Backache.
- Chronic pain.
- Delayed recovery from surgery.
- Unsuccessful symptom relief.

Teenaged and young women, the pregnant, those who self-harm, those seeking postcoital contraception and those who leave before treatment are particularly likely to be suffering domestic and sexual violence (Box 12.3).

Box 12.3 **Common ways domestic violence presents to the emergency department**

- Injury.
- Suicide/parasuicide.
- Substance/alcohol abuse.
- Psychiatric illness: depression, post-traumatic stress disorder (PTSD), anxiety, eating disorders.
- Seeking postcoital contraception, sexually transmitted disease.
- Somatisation, e.g. irritable bowel disease, headache, chronic or unexplained pain (especially pelvic and chest/breast), hyperventilation, syncope. Failure to wait/discharge against medical advice.

There is a high association between child abuse, failure to thrive, child behavioural difficulties and domestic violence in the home; up to 90% of children who live in homes where domestic violence exist witness or are involved in it. Staff members must be highly suspicious of domestic and sexual violence affecting the mother whenever a child in these categories presents.

Although clinicians should routinely maintain a high level of suspicion of abuse, some presentations are good indicators of domestic and sexual violence (Boxes 12.4 and 12.5).

Box 12.4 **Indicators of domestic violence in the emergency department**

- Delay in presentation.
- Injuries inconsistent with patient story.
- Multiple attendances, polypharmacy, multiple operations.
- Past history of intrauterine death/prematurity.
- Antidepressant use.
- Evasive, apologetic or passive patient.
- Over-vehement denial of abuse.
- Partner answering for patient.
- Non-accidental injury/behavioural difficulties in patient's children.

Box 12.5 **Case study: Jane's story**

Jane Morris presented with back pain 3 days after 'falling in the kitchen'. On x-ray she had an anterior wedge fracture of her

10th thoracic vertebra, characteristic of violent flexion. On further questioning, Jane revealed that her husband had thrown her to the floor. Jane was judged high risk because of the force required to cause this fracture. She was admitted and referred to the local MARAC.

Many general medical disorders have also been associated with past experiences of domestic and sexual violence; violence should be considered when patients present with cardiovascular disease, liver disease, chronic lung disease/smoking, cancer or osteoarthritis.

How to approach the patient

Interview the patient alone. This may call for ingenuity, particularly if the suspected abuser is present and is unwilling to leave. Strategies include interviewing the patient in x-ray or a procedure room from which the accompanying person is excluded because of 'radiation or infection control risks'. It may be necessary to admit the patient to an observation bed in order to get privacy and time for discussion. Where the patient does not speak English, use an independent translator rather than a family member or friend, who may be complicit.

Be nonjudgemental towards both the patient and the perpetrator. Believe patients and treat them with compassion and empathy. It is the rule, rather than the exception, for the patient to return to the abuser at some stage. They will be reluctant to seek help again if they feel criticised or if the perpetrator has been roundly condemned (Box 12.6).

Box 12.6 **Approach to the patient**

- Exclude partner (or other companions), interview in privacy.
- Ask direct questions gently.
- Be nonjudgmental.
- Emphasise the appropriateness of the patient's attendance.
- Discuss safety: How at risk does the patient feel? Are there weapons in the home? Are there children? Are they safe?
- Explore options: What sources of support does the patient have? What safe havens? What have they tried before? What do they want to do re legal action? Are the police involved?
- Move at the patient's own pace and nurture their right to make their own decisions.

The evidence is that over 95% of emergency department attenders welcome enquiry about violence and that only 25% of domestic and sexual violence patients disclose spontaneously (Box 12.7).

Box 12.7 **How to ask in the emergency department**

Be direct. For example, if faced with a patient with a black eye:

'I know that you have told me that you hurt yourself slipping against a door knob but, in my experience, your kind of injury is much more commonly caused by an assault than a fall. Most of these assaults happen in the home. Is this what has happened to you?'

Then wait for an answer.
If necessary, wait long enough that you begin to become uncomfortable with the silence, and then a bit longer.
Most people will say something within this time.

If abuse is denied but you are suspicious of domestic or sexual violence, record the suspicion in the notes. Even when abuse is denied, safe enquiry can in itself be therapeutically useful (Box 12.8).

Box 12.8 Case study: Dr Sue Sullivan's story

Dr Sue Sullivan, a senior emergency department doctor, was distressed when a patient who had presented with black eyes twice in a month reacted badly to being asked about domestic violence (despite it being in privacy, without being overheard) by storming out and complaining loudly to her partner and the entire waiting room, 'How dare anyone think such a thing?' and threatening legal action. In discussion with a colleague, Sue realised that her patient had acted to protect herself in two ways. She had made the abuse public and her partner now knew that people were aware of it. She had also demonstrated her complete loyalty to him.

Examination and investigations

Immediate medical and psychological care is the first priority but in all cases where domestic or sexual violence is suspected or reported, high-quality clinical records (Boxes 12.9 and 12.10) and the preservation of forensic evidence are vital (see Chapters 18 and 20). A patient who does not want to take criminal or civil action at the time they attend may still need solid evidence later for subsequent legal proceedings. If the patient does not want the police involved, record their version of events in full and verbatim (see Chapter 20). If the police will be taking a detailed statement then the clinical notes can be restricted to essential information.

Box 12.9 Documentation of injuries

- *Examine and document meticulously.*
- *Sign and date all notes.*
- Time, date, place of abuse.
- Patient's statement of perpetrator and events, including their actions after the assault.
- Witnesses.
- Injury size, pattern, age, location: note bite and fingertip marks.
- Signs of sexual abuse.
- Non-bodily evidence, e.g. torn clothing.

Box 12.10 Taking photographs

- Get written consent.
- Take high-quality photographs, both identifying the patient and detailing the injuries.
- Sign and date the back of each photograph.

- Put photographs in a sealed envelope firmly attached to the medical records, dated and labelled.
- Photographs should only be released as per usual access-to-medical-records protocols.
- Advise patient to have repeat photographs after 2–3 days, when bruising will be more evident.

Ideally, all forensic evidence should be collected by the police, forensic medical examiners or at SARCs. SARCs and most forensic medical examiners will collect evidence even when the patient does not want the police involved initially. Where a forensic medical examiner is involved, take advice before/while treating the patient. It is important that evidence is not lost, so staff members should be able to advise patients on the preservation of evidence, obtain 'early evidence' samples of urine and mouth rinse if the police have not already done so (Figure 12.1) and collect evidence when the patient does not want police involvement and there is no local SARC (Box 12.11).

Box 12.11 Evidence collection

- Wear gloves.
- Package all items separately and seal and label immediately.
- Clothing: place in paper police evidence bags (put wet clothing in an *open* plastic police evidence bag first).
- Everything else: place in plastic police evidence bags.
- Put in locked storage until collected by police.
- Maintain chain of evidence by recording every handover (sign, date and time).

Collect:

- Early evidence samples, if not done by police.
- Condoms, tampons, sanitary towels, chewing gum.
- All clothing removed.
- Debris.
- Paper sheet, trolley cover (fold the sheet/cover inwards to preserve any debris on it).
- Temporary dressings, wound and catheterisation swabs.

Sexual violence patients should not wash, wipe, clean their teeth, eat, smoke, chew gum or remove potential evidence, such as tampons or clothes. They should not urinate before the early evidence collection. If possible, patients should undress standing on a brown paper sheet; this and the paper/linen trolley cover must be preserved. Any clothing removed should be cut off in such a way that forensic evidence is not damaged, staying well clear of wound areas. Injuries such as bites that do not require immediate repair should not be cleaned, so that DNA evidence is preserved. Pelvic examination should be left to the forensic medical examiner/SARC unless there is evidence of significant injury that requires immediate treatment or examination under anaesthesia.

Investigations may include pregnancy testing to inform treatment and bloods for HIV and hepatitis B testing. If the patient is going to a SARC, these tests will be performed there.

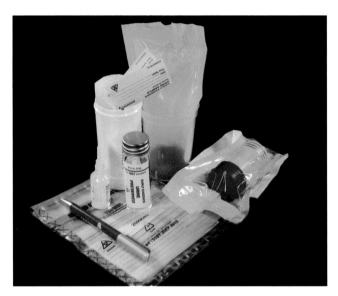

Figure 12.1 Typical early evidence kit. Source: www.scenesafe.co.uk. Reproduced with permission.

Help and advice can be sought from the forensic examiner, SARC and genitourinary medicine/sexual health teams. Useful flowcharts and forms are available at www.careandevidence.org.

Treatment, referral and follow-up

The treatment of injury and illness follows usual protocols. Where patients have suffered sexual assault, you should offer postcoital contraception where necessary and discuss prophylaxis for blood-borne viruses and bacterial sexually transmitted infections (STIs). You can obtain advice from your local SARC or genitourinary medicine/microbiology on-call. Also see Chapters 18 and 19.

Domestic violence patients should be risk-assessed and high-risk patients should be referred to the local independent domestic violence advisor (IDVA), who will work with them to increase their and their children's safety, and to a MARAC, an information-sharing meeting aimed at increasing the safety of those most at risk from domestic abuse. All information shared must be in the context of prevention and detection of crime or serious harm and must follow Caldicott principles. Referral can be made on the basis of professional serious concern or a high score (usually >14/24) on the CAADA-DASH (Coordinated Action Against Domestic Abuse & Domestic Abuse, Stalking and 'Honour'-Based Violence) risk identification checklist (see Appendix B).

Sexual violence patients can be referred to an independent sexual violence advisor (ISVA) and/or SARC and should be followed up in the local SARC or the genitourinary medicine clinic 10–14 days after the assault, or 2–3 days if given HIV post-exposure prophylaxis.

Domestic and sexual violence patients need ongoing psychosocial support; specialist domestic and sexual violence advisors or advocates, SARCs, genitourinary medicine services and the patient's GP can provide/refer to appropriate care (Box 12.12).

Box 12.12 **Treatment and referral**

- Compassion, empathy and belief.
- Treat the presenting condition.
- After sexual assault:
  - Levonelle 1.5 mg stat.
  - If >3 days post-assault, consider intrauterine contraceptive device.
  - Infection prophylaxis: hep B immunoglobulin and accelerated vaccination course if non-immune/unknown status.
  - HIV PEP within 1 hour.
  - Antibiotics: e.g. Cefixime 400 mg stat Azithromycin 1 g stat +/− Metronidazole 2 g stat.
- Risk assess: refer high-risk patients to IDVA/MARAC.
- Psychosocial support:
  - IVDA/ISDA.
  - SARC.
  - Genitourinary medicine service.
  - General practitioner.

Discharge

Abused people become disempowered. A bossy or authoritarian approach by clinicians compounds the disempowerment. Advice needs to acknowledge that the patient knows their own situation best: they may be at more risk if they leave than if they stay, they may have considerable investment in the relationship (e.g. children), they may have no financial independence and be socially isolated, they may not be psychologically in a place where they can evaluate their options.

Having explored the patient's perception of their situation, the clinician should focus on information about possible actions and sources of support. Emergency housing can be found through Refuge, the social services and in extreme cases the police. The patient can take action under both the criminal and civil law. Women's Aid and Refuge offer support both when a domestic violence survivor has left their partner and when they are staying (see Box 12.13 and Chapters 8 and 9).

Box 12.13 **Key sources of support**

Independent

- National helpline: 0808 2000 247.
- Women's Aid (survivor's handbook, directory of local domestic and sexual violence services, survivor's forum, advice for children).
- Refuge (emergency accommodation, IDVAs, outreach services, child support workers, culturally specific help).
- Rape crisis (centres providing crisis and long-term sexual violence counselling, support and advocacy).

Statutory

- GP.
- Community support unit (police).
- Family planning clinic.
- Alcohol/drug team.
- Social services.

When a domestic violence patient is returning to the abuser, you should discuss what they would do 'if things got worse, if you had to escape'; that is, an 'exit plan' (Box 12.14).

Box 12.14 Suggestions for an exit plan

Establish an alert code with your friends or family (e.g. a particular phrase during a phone conversation) and agree what they should do in response to it (e.g. call the police, come round, collect your children from school).

Ask a neighbour to call the police if they hear violence begin.

Put together an emergency bag and leave it with someone you trust. Put in the bag:

- Contact numbers for support services and personal key contacts, address book.
- Spare house and car keys.
- Medications that you or the children need.
- Enough money to get through at least a couple of days.
- A couple of days' worth of clothes and toiletries for you and your children.
- Essential legal documents, e.g. passports, visas, work permit, birth certificates, lease or mortgage details, driving licence, National Insurance number.
- Cheque book, debit/credit cards, bank books.
- Small possessions of high financial or sentimental value.
- Small toys for the children.

An alert marker should be added to adult records and medical notes can cover the violent episode fully. However, both parents have access to their children's records so, while an alert marker should be added to paediatric notes, the abused parent should be protected by keeping records of the violence separate from the child records – either as part of their own medical record or in a back-office confidential file.

Lastly, while the patient should be reassured that nothing they disclose will be shared with the abuser or any member of the public without their permission, if they or the children are judged to be at serious risk then confidentiality will need to be broken and local safeguarding procedures/referral to MARACs will have to be instigated (see Chapter 5). Every effort must be made to obtain the patient's agreement first.

Being prepared for a patient experiencing domestic or sexual violence

It is important to acquaint yourself with the resources in your department and in the local area.

In the emergency department

- Are there forensic specimen bags?
- Are there early evidence kits?
- Where are forensic specimen bags/kits kept?
- How do you take photographs? In hours/out of hours?
- Who is the MARAC link person?
- Where are the MARAC risk assessment forms kept?
- Who do you contact for HIV risk assessment/advice/post-exposure prophylaxis? In hours/out of hours?
- Is there information on key support service contacts to give patients (often credit card-sized lists of local and national contact numbers)?
- Where is the patient information kept?
- How do you refer to alcohol/drug services? In hours/out of hours?
- What support is there for staff members? How do you access it?

In the area

- Is there a local SARC? If yes, how do you contact them?
- Is there an IDVA available to the department? If yes, how do you contact them?
- Is there a local MARAC?
- How do you contact the forensic medical examiner?
- How do you contact the community support unit?
- How do you contact social services?

Further reading

Department of Health (2012) *'Striking the Balance': Practical Guidance on the Application of Caldicott Guardian Principles to Domestic Violence and MARACs (Multi Agency Risk Assessment Conferences)*, http://www.dh.gov.uk/en/Publicationsandstatistics/Publications/PublicationsPolicyAnd Guidance/DH_133589 (last accessed 12 February 2014).

Web sites

Broken Rainbow, www.broken-rainbow.org.uk (last accessed 12 February 2014).
CAADA, www.caada.org.uk (last accessed 12 February 2014).
Care and Evidence, www.careandevidence.org (last accessed 12 February 2014).
The Havens, www.thehavens.org.uk (last accessed 12 February 2014).
Rape Crisis, www.rapecrisis.org.uk (last accessed 12 February 2014).
Refuge, www.refuge.org.uk (last accessed 12 February 2014).
Royal College of Physicians Faculty of Forensic and Legal Medicine, http://fflm.ac.uk (last accessed 12 February 2014).
Victim Support, www.victimsupport.org.uk (last accessed 12 February 2014).
Womens Aid, www.womensaid.org.uk (last accessed 12 February 2014).

CHAPTER 13

Elder Abuse

Finbarr C. Martin

Department of Geriatrics, Guys and St Thomas' NHS Trust, UK

OVERVIEW

- Elders may be abused by partners, family, neighbours and carers
- Neglect is the commonest form of abuse
- In the community, the abuser is often an individual with problems related to mental health, relationships or financial security
- Supportive care planning reduces the chance of abuse by informal care givers
- In our ageing society, health care staff will need the skills and attitudes required to meet the needs of older people

What is elder abuse and how much is there?

The definition adopted by the World Health Organization is given in Box 13.1. It concerns the experience of older people within relationships with family, friends or formal carers, but not assault by strangers or others, which would be regarded in law in the same way as it would for other citizens.

Box 13.1 **World Health Organization definition of elder abuse**

'A single or repeated act or lack of appropriate action, occuring within any relationship where there is an expectation of trust, which causes harm or distress to an older person'.

There are five recognised categories of elder abuse:

- **Physical**: e.g. assault such as physical hitting, rough handling during care provision, unreasonable restraint, forced feeding, deliberate overmedication.
- **Psychological**: e.g. insults, shouting, humiliation, forced isolation.
- **Financial**: e.g. unauthorised use of funds, selling of property, forced taking of 'loans'.
- **Sexual**: e.g. sexual contact without consent, including lack of capacity to consent.
- **Neglect**: e.g. denial of necessary reasonable care or access to care.

The UK study of Abuse and Neglect of Older People (commissioned by Comic Relief and the Department of Health; O'Keeffe *et al.*, 2007) reported in 2007 that 2.6% of people aged 66 and over living in private households had experienced mistreatment involving a family member, close friend or care worker during the past year (see Biggs *et al.*, 2013). This equates to nearly a quarter of a million individuals in the UK. When broadened to include acts of mistreatment by neighbours or acquaintances, the prevalence increases to 4%.

Neglect is the commonest form of abuse, followed by financial, psychological, physical and sexual abuse, and it is not uncommon to experience two or more types of mistreatment together. Women are more likely to be in relationships of dependency in very old age and are three times more likely to report abuse. People on previous lower incomes and in rented accommodation are far more likely to be abused than higher-income owner-occupiers.

Who are the abusers?

Overall, a third of cases of mistreatment are by neighbours and acquaintances, a third by partners and the rest by other family members (including carers). Most abusers (80%) are men. An estimated two-thirds of cases of abuse occur in the elder's home and the remainder in various institutional settings (i.e. by paid carers), but direct comparative surveys have not been undertaken. Abuse can happen in any context and the reasons behind it are complex.

Why does it happen?

Abuse is more likely in the context of poor long-term family relationships, and there may be a past history of family violence. It may be associated with the carer's inability to cope or consistently provide the care needed. But this is usually not related to the nature of the caring provided, or even factors often associated with care giver stress such as the behavioural challenges of dementia. More often, it is associated with physical or mental health problems

---

ABC of Domestic and Sexual Violence, First Edition.
Edited by Susan Bewley and Jan Welch.
© 2014 John Wiley & Sons, Ltd. Published 2014 by John Wiley & Sons, Ltd.

in the carer, particularly depression and alcohol abuse in men (see Box 13.2).

Box 13.2 Case study

Mrs Antony is a frail woman of 84 years of age. She is brought into the emergency department by ambulance following a fall at home, and admitted to a medical ward with a diagnosis of delirium probably precipitated by urosepsis. The nursing staff finds her to be unwashed, with evidence of faecal soiling. Her son, John, a single man, who called the ambulance, arrives a little later with her tablets. He is unkempt himself. The next day, further collateral history is obtained by the medical staff.

- What else might be going on with the mother?
- What else might be going on with the son?
- What else do you need to know?

Mrs Antony is ill, and needs careful assessment and differential diagnosis (of fall and delirium). She may have further collateral or underlying diagnoses. Her son may have medical, mental or social difficulties himself that interfere with his ability to care for his mother. It is important to collect information from old notes, previous admissions and other sources.

Mrs Antony is discharged home the next day with planned input from the community rapid response team. Realising that their involvement could be perceived as an intrusion, or even as criticism of his abilities, the team plans to include John in their efforts, and simultaneously to appraise his need for advice and support.

- Who else might be involved in the wider team?

There are many sources of information and help, including the GP, district nurse, social services, private care agencies, other relatives, friends and neighbours.

Unfortunately, Mrs Antony's daughter died 6 months ago, and John does not allow the team in for their second, evening visit. The social worker reports that he previously stopped regular care input from a care agency after 2 weeks. This event raises several possibilities. He may have problems such as alcohol dependency that he is concealing by restricting access. He may be dependent on his mother's resources and fear that payment for care will financially cripple him. His mother may well have been protectively complicit in such behaviour in the past, despite its negative impact on her. But if she has developed dementia and lost the mental capacity to appreciate her increasing vulnerability then protective action may be needed to prevent neglect due to denial of access to essential care. This is a complex situation that requires patience and a team-based approach. There may be a need to balance ethical principles of confidentiality with the need to enhance Mrs Anthony's autonomy. Procrastination should be avoided and the potential need for urgent intervention must be kept in mind.

Neglect may occur through ignorance or a lack of skills and available external support or supervision. Like other abuse, it may be either premeditated or (more commonly) opportunistically perpetrated. Hostilities of all sorts, including prejudices, may play a part. Abuse in institutional settings is briefly mentioned later in the chapter.

The doctor's role

In line with other professionals, doctors can play an important role in anticipating, preventing, identifying and reacting to the presence or suspicion of abuse.

Anticipate

Awareness of the prevalence, type and context is important. Identifying stress in caring relationships, mental health problems on the part of the carer or dementia and severe physical dependency on the part of the cared-for person should always include consideration that arrangements may break down and cause abuse.

Prevent

Care planning for older people with complex needs could do much to ensure that those involved are given the advice and support necessary to avoid crisis situations. This includes assessment of any informal carer's attitudes and skills. Sensitive enquiry about stresses associated with caring and even hostility that has not translated into abusive actions should be gently elicited.

Identify

There are no features on physical or mental health examination which are pathognomonic of abuse. Screening assessments by either enquiry or examination have not so far been shown useful.

Detection in community care

Suspicion of abuse may be raised when providing community health or social care or when reviewing progress or care plans, by a lack of cooperation in making arrangements or seeking routine information, broken agreements concerning access, evasion at the doorstep and so on. Neglect may be obvious, but other abuse less so. Observing behaviour, either when the older person is alone or when they are in the company of the potential abuser, is important.

Detection in the clinical setting

Documentation and investigation of clinical events such as falls, fractures, aspiration pneumonia, pressure sores and bruises is necessary because the causes of these may include abusive behaviour or neglect. The general appearance of being cared for or neglected is important. Obviously, evidence of bruises, lacerations and so on should be noted, but more subtle clinical events might include recurrent urinary infections and unusually sited or shaped bruises or abrasions.

Evidence of sexual abuse may take the form of rectal or vaginal bleeding or (rarely) vaginal discharge suggesting infection.

Psychological abuse is more likely to occur alongside physical or financial abuse. Common examples include terrorisation through real or imagined threats and control over access to visitors or telephone calls. Mental health examination, including of behaviours, is important in identifying potential psychological abuse.

An older person's seeming hesitant to talk openly, providing implausible stories for injuries, being angry or upset without good cause or otherwise displaying fear or withdrawal is noteworthy.

React

If concerns exist in either setting then local procedures should be followed. Broadly speaking, all four nations of the UK take a similar approach, although in Scotland the protection policy and procedures based on the Adult Support and Protection (Scotland) Act 2007 do not use the term 'abuse' but rather 'harm' and 'adults at risk of harm'. In 2011, the Older People's Commissioner for Wales produced *Protection of Older People in Wales: A Guide to the Law* to guide the responsible interagency regional and local bodies. The Northern Ireland office created an adult safeguarding partnership in 2010. In England there are local adult safeguarding teams, led by local authority social services.

It is important that doctors work alongside other colleagues in the multidisciplinary team to record, discuss and plan a response to real or potential abuse. In addition to taking a careful general history and a collateral and clinical examination, it is important to interview patients alone with direct but unforceful enquiries about physical injuries and marks of restraint or neglect, recording carefully the details of the nature, frequency and severity of events.

It is not the doctor's job to act as policeman or accuser, and he or she may not be the best person to fill this role. Information may not be given freely, as the older person may have reasons to collude in or to conceal abuse. In such cases, it is important to assess mental capacity, as consent for activities, including financial transactions, may be invalid.

Taking a history from a potential abuser is a job for an experienced person. It requires training to avoid confrontation and to consider the older person's carer's understanding and role.

Sexual abuse is a crime regardless of the age of the victim and suspicions of this must be accompanied by good evidence gathering; it is important while providing care and comfort not to take actions that remove or compromise evidence.

Neglect in institutions

Recent research has highlighted that members of hospital staff who are surprised to find themselves looking after older people with multiple illnesses are less likely to meet their needs adequately. Unfortunately the public discussions about hospitals being unsuitable places for older people may make health care staff think such individuals will not be in their care, but 70% of acute general hospital beds will be occupied by older people, many of whom will need to remain in hospital due to the effects of several conditions.

Therefore, understanding and meeting the needs of older people is core business for the NHS, and failure to prepare our workforce accordingly will lead to neglect.

Media reports of neglect or abuse in care homes rightly raise public concern but there are no reliable estimates of incidence. Regulation plays a part in promoting good care, but so does a well trained and supported workforce with equitable access to NHS services. Public policy and practice in the UK do not yet provide this.

Further reading

Biggs, S., Erens, B., Doyle, M., Hall, J. & Sanchez, M. (2013) Abuse and neglect of older people: secondary analysis of UK prevalence study, http://www.natcen.ac.uk/media/20824/abuse-neglect-older-people.pdf (last accessed 12 February 2014).

British Geriatrics Society (2005) Abuse of older people, http://www.bgs.org.uk/index.php/topresources/publicationfind/goodpractice/370-elderabuse (last accessed 12 February 2014).

Daly, J.M., Merchant, M.L. & Jogerst, G.J. (2011) Elder abuse research: a systematic review. *Journal of Elder Abuse & Neglect*, **23**(4), 348–365, http://dx.doi.org/10.1080/08946566.2011.608048 (last accessed 12 February 2014).

Department of Health (2011) Statement of government policy on adult safeguarding, http://www.dh.gov.uk/en/Publicationsandstatistics/Publications/PublicationsPolicyAndGuidance/DH_126748 (last accessed 12 February 2014).

Lachs, M.S. & Pillimer, K. (2004) Elder abuse. *Lancet*, **364**, 1263–1272.

McDonald, L., Beaulieu, M., Harbison, J., Hirst, S., Lowenstein, A., Podnieks, E. & Wahl, J. (2012) Abuse of older adults: what we know, what we need to know. *Journal of Elder Abuse & Neglect*, **24**(2), 138–160, http://dx.doi.org/10.1080/08946566.2011.646512 (last accessed 12 February 2014).

O'Keeffe, M., Hills, A., Doyle, M., McCreadie, C., Scholes, S., Constantine, R., Tinker, A., Manthorpe, J., Biggs, S. & Erens, B.; prepared for Comic Relief and the Department of Health (2007) UK study of abuse and neglect of older people: prevalence survey report, http://webarchive.nationalarchives.gov.uk/20130107105354/http://www.dh.gov.uk/en/Publicationsandstatistics/Publications/PublicationsPolicyAndGuidance/DH_076197 (last accessed 12 February 2014).

Web site

Action on Elder Abuse, www.elderabuse.org.uk (last accessed 12 February 2014).

PANICOA (Prevention of Abuse and Neglect in the Institutional Care of Older Adults), http://www.panicoa.org.uk (last accessed 12 February 2014).

CHAPTER 14

The Dental Team

Tim Newton[1] and Rasha Al Dabaan[2]

[1]Dental Institute, King's College London, UK
[2]Department of Pediatric Dentistry and Orthodontics, King Saud University, College of Dentistry, Saudi Arabia

---

OVERVIEW

- Dentists have a professional duty of care regarding abuse, neglect and violence
- Physical abuse often manifests in head injuries
- Dentists can be professionally isolated
- Training and procedures are needed to overcome this

Context of dental consultation

General dental practitioners (GDPs) have a professional duty of care to identify and respond to domestic abuse, neglect and sexual violence when observed in their patients. Furthermore, the dental team may be ideally placed to detect some forms of violent crime; physical abuse often manifests as an assault on the person's head and face, and such injuries are likely to present at dental practices. Despite this, a number of perceived barriers exist to the dental team's becoming involved in protecting vulnerable patients. These include a lack of knowledge of the area, the isolation of dentistry from other health care providers, the perceptions of dentists regarding their role in protection of vulnerable patients and a disproportionate focus in dental research on child abuse.

Dentists' knowledge and skills

One of the greatest problems is a lack of knowledge of the signs of abuse and the mechanisms for dealing with instances of abuse when identified. Many GDPs also have little confidence in dealing competently with domestic and sexual violence. Since 2005, mandatory training in the protection of vulnerable patients has been introduced as part of the core continuing professional development requirements for continued registration with the General Dental Council.

GDPs are often isolated from other health care professionals and from people involved in social services or law enforcement. It is thus more difficult for GDPs to consult informally with others about their concerns or to learn about protection mechanisms through experience or observation.

Dentists may not feel that recognising and reporting abuse is their responsibility. In the case of reporting domestic violence, they may feel that such actions will have detrimental consequences for themselves and their practice and will involve them in complex social and legal issues.

It is also true that dental research in the UK has given considerable attention to orofacial signs of physical abuse in children, whereas far less attention has been paid to domestic violence, emotional abuse and sexual abuse.

Threshold of suspicion

The neglect of domestic violence and the abuse of vulnerable adults in the mainstream UK dental literature suggest that these are areas that should be targeted in future educational programmes for dentists, as they will see patient with problems (see Box 14.1). As with child abuse, the recognition and management of domestic violence and the abuse of vulnerable adults are discussed more fully in the dental literature emanating from the USA.

Box 14.1 **Case scenario**

A 34-year-old mother attends the dental surgery accompanied by her rather clingy 7-year-old son on a Tuesday morning. She complains of pain from a broken tooth in her upper-left jaw and a clicking noise and pain coming from her temporomandibular joint. She has a healing bruise under her left eye, which is only partially masked with make-up. Looking at the notes, you see she has a frequent history of missed appointments and problems in paying for previous treatment. On examination, she shows signs of pain and has a broken crown on her upper-left lateral incisor. She appears to be guarding her arms, which you cannot see because she is wearing long sleeves.

Concerns

1 There is obvious evidence of injury, and possibly additional injuries.
2 The mother may be financially dependent upon her partner, both for treatment and for money more generally.
3 The child is at risk in a home where there is domestic violence.
4 The boy is accompanying his mother and thus is not in primary school.
5 There is a history of missed dental appointments.

ABC of Domestic and Sexual Violence, First Edition.
Edited by Susan Bewley and Jan Welch.
© 2014 John Wiley & Sons, Ltd. Published 2014 by John Wiley & Sons, Ltd.

Possible actions

- Discuss your findings and concerns with the patient and explain the treatment needed.
- Deliver treatment in the short term for the injuries and plan long-term management of the broken dentition.
- Keep clear and accurate documentation in the clinical records of the extra- and intra-oral findings, as well as of any discussions that take place in the surgery, using the patient's language as much as possible.
- Discuss concerns with a senior colleague as appropriate.
- Enquire whether the child or any of his siblings are registered at the local child protection register held by children's social services within the area in which they reside.
- Arrange for recall appointments.
- Contact the local safeguarding team.

Box 14.2 shows 'red flags' for abuse and violence that might present in the dental consultation. The principles of sensitive questioning and referral are similar to those described in other chapters (see for example Chapters 3 and 7).

Box 14.2 **'Red flags' for abuse and violence presenting in the dental consultation**

- Bruise on the cheek (leaving finger marks and often on the left side of the face).
- Bruise on the ear (may be a result of pinch marks).
- Petechia or ecchymosis of the mucosa and soft or hard palates.
- Discoloured teeth from previous trauma.
- Fractured, displaced or avulsed teeth.
- Facial bone/jaw fracture.
- Malocclusion as a result of fracture to maxilla or mandible.
- Burns (chemical, scalding liquids).
- Bite marks.
- Inappropriate clothes for the weather, e.g. a loose sweater in hot weather.
- Aggression/hostility.
- Lack of social responsiveness/passivity.
- Detachment.
- Anxiety/depression.
- Challenging behaviour.
- Poor attention span.
- Low self-esteem.
- Substance abuse.

Ultimately, it is the professional responsibility of all GDPs to act in the best interests of their patients. This means ensuring that all members of the dental team are trained in the recognition and management of abuse and that procedures are in place to make the dental surgery a safe place for all patients to attend (see Box 14.3).

Box 14.3 **What should dentists do?**

- Find out about abuse and violence.
- Provide confidential consultation.
- Be able to ask questions sensitively (see Chapter 7).
- Empathise.
- Document (as records may be required for future civil or criminal actions).
- Advise about sources of help and local resources.
- Develop policy around adult and child protection.

Further reading

Golder, M. (1995) Non-accidental injury in children. *Dental Update*, **22**, 75-81.

Johnson, T., Boccia, A. & Strayer, M. (2001) Elder abuse and neglect: detection, reporting, and intervention. *Special Care in Dentistry*, **21**, 141–146.

Sinha, S., Acharya, P., Jafar, H., Bower, E., Harrison, V. & Newton, T. (2005) *The Management of Abuse: A Resource Manual for the Dental Team*. Stephen Hancocks, London.

CHAPTER 15

Mental Health Services

Eleanor Turner Moss[1] and Louise M. Howard[2]

[1] Barts and The London School of Medicine and Dentistry, Queen Mary University of London, UK
[2] Institute of Psychiatry, King's College London, UK

OVERVIEW

- Domestic and sexual violence are both common in people seen in mental health services, with a higher prevalence in women
- All mental disorders (including substance use disorders) are associated with an increased risk of being a victim of violence. Women with physical disabilities and learning disabilities are also at increased risk
- Domestic and sexual violence may lead to development of mental health problems and/or exacerbation of existing symptoms. Symptoms decrease and psychological therapies are more effective when abuse stops
- Most violence is not detected by health professionals; they do not feel confident in asking and victims fear the potential consequences of disclosure
- Health professionals must be able to ask about experiences of violence, be familiar with local procedures and be ready to respond appropriately if violence is disclosed, with special consideration for the vulnerabilities of the mentally ill

---

Headlines

- Domestic violence is a common hidden problem for women attending mental health services and is a major cause of mental ill health globally.
- Poor mental health produces 73%, and substance abuse 22%, of the total disease burden of domestic violence in women aged 18–44 years.
- The prevalence of any adult lifetime partner violence among psychiatric inpatients ranges from 16 to 94% among women and from 18 to 48% among men. This is often associated with prior childhood abuse.
- Identification of and response to domestic and sexual violence experienced by mental health service users is suboptimal. Currently only 10–30% is detected by health professionals.

Myths and myth busters

- Mental health service users are often perceived as perpetrators of violence but they are actually more likely to be victims.
- Internationally, there are no consistent demographic associations with interpersonal violence (including age, ethnicity and number of children) other than relative poverty (see Figure 15.1).
- The majority of service users do not mind being asked about violence when the enquiry is justified, introduced as routine and made by a supportive professional whom they trust.
- Emotional abuse is more damaging than physical abuse for a victim's mental health.

Typical presentations

The presence of any mental disorder is itself a possible indicator of violence (see Boxes 15.1 and 15.2). Examples of presentations of related mental illness include:

- A middle-aged woman presenting to her GP with depression and old bruising.
- A young woman with learning disabilities in obvious distress but unable to state what the problem is.
- A mother with schizophrenia presenting with exacerbation of psychotic symptoms.
- A young man with panic attacks and symptoms of hyper-arousal.
- A woman in A&E who has made a suicide attempt and has a history of self-harm.
- A mother with back pain and a recent worsening of alcohol abuse.

Box 15.1 **Case study**

Sarah Jackson, a 38-year-old woman who is currently experiencing a psychotic breakdown, tells you that she is experiencing hallucinations and is finding it difficult to cope. Sarah has attended with her partner, who asks to sit in on the meeting; he tells you she has 'gone mad again' and does not allow her much time to speak. However, she does disclose she is drinking more alcohol than usual.

Suggestions

- Ask to see her alone (without her partner present) as is routine.
- Ask about her relationship, including specific questions about physical, sexual and emotional abuse.

ABC of Domestic and Sexual Violence, First Edition.
Edited by Susan Bewley and Jan Welch.
© 2014 John Wiley & Sons, Ltd. Published 2014 by John Wiley & Sons, Ltd.

- Give her a key message (see Box 15.3).
- Offer information about key services.

Box 15.2 **Case study**

Anna Turner, a 40-year-old, has attended a number of times this year. She moved to the UK 2 years ago with her husband and has one child, now 8 months old. Anna speaks reasonable English and always attends appointments with her young child. She has recurrent depressive episodes and regularly reports difficulties coping with day-to-day life. She has frequent headaches and today has a black eye.

Suggestions

- Ask about her injury.
- Ask about other experiences of domestic violence.
- Give her a key message (see Box 15.3).
- Check whether she is safe to return to her home.
- Offer information about key services and discuss options available to her.

Clinical tips

- Always remember violence as a potential trigger in an acute presentation or exacerbation of mental illness.
- Do not assume that just because patients have paranoid delusions what they are saying is necessarily false.

- In thought disorder, patients may not be able to give a clear and coherent history or description of violence.
- Request an independent interpreter and ask them to sign a confidentiality agreement. Never let a partner, family member, child or friend translate.
- Even one question on domestic violence can increase disclosure rates by 10%.
- Disclosure is a process, so ask on more than one occasion.
- Assess the direct risk from the abuser but also the risk of self-harm and suicide.
- Cases are often complicated, so do get clinical supervision. Discuss cases with a senior clinician and specialist services.

Complicating factors

- Women experiencing domestic violence are more than six times more likely to misuse or develop dependence on alcohol and drugs.
- There will be situations in which it is not appropriate to ask about domestic or sexual violence, such as when a patient is agitated, psychotic or acutely disturbed. It is still important to ask when the patient is less disturbed so that a full assessment can be carried out.
- Children are at risk even just from witnessing violence to others. Be sure to assess risk to all children and other family members.
- Be cautious when receiving a collateral history from a potential abuser. Do not assume their account is accurate and be wary about sharing patient details or plans.
- Most domestic violence homicides occur at the point of separation.

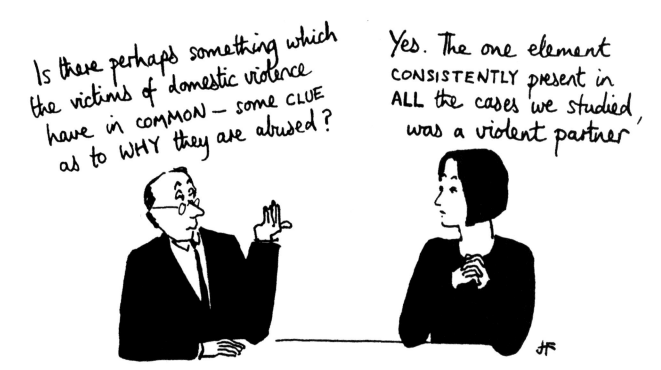

Figure 15.1 What do victims of domestic violence have in common? Source: www.jackyfleming.co.uk. Copyright © 2013 Jacky Fleming. Reproduced with permission.

How to ask

Most patients do not mind being asked about violence when it is explained that enquiry is routine (see Chapter 7), the problem is common (one in four women experience domestic or sexual violence at some point) and you can help refer them to expert services. It is vital that a patient feels supported and able to trust their health professional.

Consultations must be private and confidential. Explain where there may be mandatory reporting (for instance if there are safeguarding concerns around the patient or children). Victims may not be able speak openly while their partner or family members are present. Ensure interpreters are independent and not from the patient's community. As with other consultations, start with open questions and then move on to more closed, specific questions about violence.

An opening approach might be: 'Who's at home?' 'How are things at home?' 'What happens when there are arguments at home?'

More specifically, you might say: 'Many people I see with these sorts of symptoms have experienced domestic violence or sexual violence. Is someone hurting you or threatening you?'

If they hesitate, you could say: 'I ask because I am concerned for the safety of all my patients. I want to find out if you need information or support. I will not tell your family or partner about what you say.'

If the patient admits they have been frightened or hurt, you need to document the type of abuse suffered. Ask about physical, psychological (including emotional and financial) and sexual abuse, remembering that each group overlaps with and compounds the impact of the others. It is best to phrase questions in terms of the behaviour of the perpetrator:

- Has [your partner/a relative] ever:
  ○ kicked, punched, pushed, grabbed or tried to choke or strangle you?
  ○ tried to hurt the children?
  ○ called you insulting names, made you feel small or insisted on what you wear?
  ○ made it difficult for you to see friends/family or leave the house?
  ○ forced you into sex even though you don't want to?

If the patient answers 'No', respect their response. Do not pressure patients to disclose violence or assume that a patient is being abused any more than you would assume that they are not. However, note any nonverbal signs such as hesitation or fear in the patient and observe their interactions and relationships, such as whether the partner's behaviour seems overly protective or controlling. Where violence is denied, the Department of Health recommends documenting 'violence not disclosed'.

A nonjudgmental, comforting relationship in which you validate what the patient is saying will help facilitate disclosure. Disclosure is a process, so make sure you ask more than once. Make sure the patient is aware of the information and support available and how to access them. You can give information 'for a friend'. Be ready to assist a woman in increasing her own safety and that of her children where necessary.

What to do after disclosure

Assure the patient that you hear and care (see Box 15.3).

Box 15.3 **Key messages that mental health service users want to hear**

- You are not alone and it is not your fault.
- What you have said is helpful and important.
- People with mental health problems have the right to be safe.
- Domestic and sexual violence can affect mental health negatively.
- Safety at home is a priority.
- There is help available.
- A good father does not put his children at risk.
- Domestic violence and sexual violence are against the law.

Assess risk and check immediate safety

Your patient may need to make an emergency decision on the risk of immediate harm to herself or her children. This is an important opportunity for the patient to identify worrying patterns (such as recent escalation of violence) of which she may not have been fully aware (see Box 15.4). Ensure the patient has the capacity to make decisions and include risk assessment for self-harm or suicide. Your team will need to decide if there is a need for immediate assistance.

Box 15.4 **Potential questions by which to ascertain immediate harm**

- Is it safe for you to go home?
- Where is [the abuser]?
- What are you afraid might happen?
- What has [the abuser] threatened?
- Have there been threats to the children?
- Is there somewhere safe you can go?

Most domestic violence homicides of women occur at or around the point of separation. It is crucial to involve specialist support services in careful discussion and planning, taking the patient's fears seriously. These are often complicated cases, so do get clinical supervision and discuss matters with a senior clinician.

Document

Writing down what the patient told you is an important aspect of treatment (see Chapter 20). It shows you are listening and the notes may be important in criminal proceedings or injunctions and in providing evidence for access to housing and welfare rights. Sensitive information should not be included in letters or reports that might be seen by the perpetrator or a family member.

Offer referral to services

You may want to consider referral for psychological therapy if symptoms persist once the situation has improved. Individual cognitive behaviour therapy (CBT) treatment for women with post-traumatic stress disorder (PTSD) who are no longer experiencing violence is associated with significant improvements in psychological outcomes (see Chapter 4).

Women with severe mental disorders find it difficult to access refuges despite efforts to reduce their exclusion from mainstream services. They access domestic violence services at a late stage and may have chaotic lives and struggle to live within a structured environment. A crisis house may be more suitable.

Making links and arrangements with local outreach services is recommended (see Chapters 8 and 9). This will ensure that you both understand what services the other can provide for victims of domestic violence with mental health problems and can develop an effective partnership (see Box 15.5).

Box 15.5 **Case study**

Theresa Clarke is a 35-year-old woman diagnosed with schizophrenia. She is unmarried and has no children. She has recently ended a relationship with a younger man who had taken her sickness benefit and accused her of being unattractive. She has since been stalked by him and has sometimes allowed him into her flat to avoid being abused in public. This has often resulted in physical and sexual assault. She presents to her community nurse stating that she is frightened and wants to move away. She believes his violence is getting worse and that he may kill her. She has not contacted the police as she does not think she will be believed; the ex-partner has said he will tell them she is mad. She is becoming significantly depressed and paranoid about other people, including having delusions of reference when walking in her local shopping mall.

- The nurse contacts the local domestic violence helpline but they state they cannot find a bed at a women's refuge for her.
- Although Theresa believes this is because of her diagnosis of bipolar disorder, the domestic violence advisor suggests joint support. With the domestic violence service and her nurse both supporting her, she obtains safe accommodation.
- Her mental state is regularly reviewed with her local mental health team in order to disentangle the psychotic features in her mental state from real revictimisation she is experiencing.
- Her mood stabiliser is increased.
- Her mental state improves over the following few weeks.

Theresa is also supported in reporting her experiences to the police; several months later the abuser is sentenced to 5 years in prison and a history of similar stalking and abuse of other women emerges in court.

Consider safeguarding issues and safeguarding referral

Vulnerable adults

The Department of Health defines a vulnerable adult as 'anyone who is, or may be, in need of community services by reason of mental health or other disabilities, age or illness and who is unable to take care of themselves or protect themselves against harm or exploitation'. Key principles have been developed for work with vulnerable adults: empowerment, protection, prevention, proportionality, partnership, transparency and accountability.

It is important to determine whether a patient has capacity or not. If they are lacking capacity then the Mental Capacity Act 2005 must be used. It may be necessary to override confidentiality to ensure a vulnerable adult is protected. Decisions must be made on a fair and objective assessment of individual needs.

For victims of domestic violence being treated for severe mental disorder under a Section of the Mental Health Act, staff should be particularly strict about confidentiality. Where the nearest relative is identified as an abuser, displacement must be considered. This can be arranged through the hospital's Mental Health Act office.

Vulnerable children

In families where there is domestic violence, children witness three-quarters of abuse and half of these children are themselves abused. The Adoption and Children Act 2002 identifies 'living with and witnessing domestic violence' as a source of 'significant harm' for children, causing cognitive, psychological, social and educational impairments.

Local child safeguarding guidelines must be followed. Supporting the nonabusive parent to be safe can be the most effective form of child protection (see Box 15.6). The legal obligation to protect children and follow guidelines should be explained to the mother. Discuss with a senior professional whether the risk to the child supersedes confidentiality and whether referral to social services might be necessary.

Box 15.6 **Case study**

Estelle Robinson is a 29-year-old woman with a 6–month-old baby. She has a long history of depression and witnessed domestic violence as a child in her family home. The father of her baby is emotionally and physically abusive to her. Although they do not live together, she wants to break off all contact, which is difficult as she needs financial support for the baby. She is worried that if she contacts the police her baby will be removed from her because of her history of depression. She tells you, her doctor, about her ex-partner's behaviour at the end of an appointment in the outpatient clinic.

What you can do

- Check whether she and the baby are safe to return to her home.
- Offer information about key services and discuss options available to her, including supporting her in reporting the father's behaviour to children and families social services and the police.
- Offer increased outpatient follow-up.

Consider referral to a MARAC

Multi-agency risk assessment conferences (MARACs) are meetings between statutory and voluntary sector organisations. The majority occur monthly. Information about domestic violence victims at high risk of harm is shared and plans to protect and support victims and their children are drawn up. Specific guidance on referral procedures is available through local domestic violence coordinators or agencies (see Chapter 9).

Staff well being

Remember your own mental well being. Don't take too much on and do offload to colleagues. Talk through what you were able to offer the patient and how this could have been improved. Contact occupational health or counselling services if you need further support.

Further reading

Campbell, J., Laughon, K. & Woods, A. (2006) Impact of intimate partner abuse on physical and mental health: how does it present in clinical practice? In: Roberts, G., Hegarty, K. & Feder, G. (eds) *Intimate Partner Abuse and Health Professionals: New Approaches to Domestic Violence*. Elsevier, pp. 43–60.

Heru, A.M. (2007) Intimate partner violence: treating abuser and abused. *Advances in Psychiatric Treatment*, **13**, 376–383, http://apt.rcpsych.org /content/13/5/376.full (last accessed 12 February 2014).

Howard, L.M. (2012) Domestic violence: its relevance to psychiatry. *Advances in Psychiatric Treatment*, **18**, 129–136.

Howard, L., Feder, G. & Agnew-Davies, R. (2013) *Domestic Violence and Mental Health*. Royal College of Psychiatrists, London.

Oram, S., Trevillion, K., Feder, G. & Howard, L.M. (2013) The prevalence of domestic violence experienced by mental health service users. *British Journal of Psychiatry*, **202**, 94–99, doi:10.1192/bjp.bp.112.109934.

Rose, D., Trevillion, K., Woodall, A., Morgan, C., Feder, G. & Howard, L. (2011) Barriers and facilitators of disclosures of domestic violence by mental health service users: qualitative study. *British Journal of Psychiatry*, **198**, 189–194.

Trevillion, K., Oram, S., Feder, G. & Howard, L.M. (2012) Experiences of domestic violence and mental disorders: a systematic review and meta-analysis. *PLoS ONE*, **7**(12), e51740, doi:10.1371/journal.pone. 0051740.

CHAPTER 16

Women's, Reproductive and Sexual Health Services

Maureen Dalton

SARC Commissioning, South West, UK

OVERVIEW

- At least one in four women are victims of abuse during their lifetime
- Victims become heavier users of the health service
- Consider the possibility of current or past abuse at every opportunity for any woman in front of you
- You can provide a confidential, trusting, women-centred space
- Such spaces will lead to diagnostic accuracy and sensitivity of relationships to improve

Introduction

Women who are victims of domestic abuse, sexual assault and previous sexual abuse are commonly seen in clinics in women's, reproductive and sexual health services, whether they be obstetrics, gynaecology, family planning, termination of pregnancy or genitourinary medicine clinics.

Start a mini mental checklist as you read the referral letter, scan the notes and take the history.

- Does the patient have thick notes and/or has she attended many departments?
- Does she have a history of mental health problems or drug or alcohol abuse?
- Does she have a high 'did not attend' rate?
- Has she 'discharged against medical advice'?
- Does she show certain obstetric and gynaecology presenting complaints (see later in chapter)?

As the risk factors mount up, this should increase suspicion that the woman may have been abused or has other complicated social or stigmatising problems.

If your suspicion has been raised, check the privacy of the area in which you are seeing the patient (Box 16.1).

Box 16.1 **Checking that you are in a 'safe space' for a private conversation (all medical practice)**

- *Is the room/cubicle soundproof?* Curtains are not! You must see the patient in a soundproof room to protect her privacy. If she is on a ward, insist on using a *soundproof* treatment room.
- *Is the window open?* If so, close it. Sound carries and the patient's abuser or a relative of the abuser may be outside. We can all recognise friends' and families' voices over those of others, and from further away.
- *Check your concerns*: It may be appropriate to share your concerns with any other professional who is in the room.
- *As the patient walks into the room, is she alone?* If her partner is with her, is he clearly dominant/overbearing? Does he take the seat near you and leave her sitting to the side? Does he answer all the questions? Does she constantly look at him to check her answers? Does he make you feel uncomfortable? Does he avoid eye contact? We can pick up signals subconsciously; these instincts should not be dismissed out of hand.
- *Has a member of the family offered to translate?* You must use independent translators (preferably an anonymous one via telephone. If a patient comes from a country that has only a small community in your area, the translator may still know her even if they are employed independently).
- *See the woman alone for some part of the consultation*: Even having her mother or sister there will inhibit a discussion about domestic or sexual abuse.
- *Try to examine the woman alone*: If this fails, say you want to check her urine. Send the nurse or chaperone off with her and explain that while separated, she needs to be asked.
- *It may be appropriate to ask the partner to leave*: Say that while you appreciate the support they are giving, sometimes patients like the extra confidentiality of being seen alone for a few minutes with the doctor. Or say, 'it's a standard of care, and professional responsibility, to ensure a short confidential time alone'. Reassure the companion(s) that you will bring them back before you explain what you want to do about her presenting problem.
- *Having a 'red spot system' in all toilets may also be useful*: This involves putting a notice on the inside door of the toilet asking if a woman is a victim of abuse and would like to talk to someone about it, and pinning some red spots on the door. The victim can then put a red spot on her urine sample if she wants to talk to someone at a safe time.

ABC of Domestic and Sexual Violence, First Edition.
Edited by Susan Bewley and Jan Welch.
© 2014 John Wiley & Sons, Ltd. Published 2014 by John Wiley & Sons, Ltd.

- *If you cannot get private time, do not endanger the patient or yourself*: If the partner objects, this should raise further suspicion. Wait for another opportunity or pass your concerns on to the next carer, the midwife or the GP.
- *Asking about abuse does not take long*: You do have time. A video of the author, for a research project in an antenatal clinic that had nothing to do with abuse, timed how long it took to ask and receive an answer. On average, it took 26 seconds before the conversation could move on to other clinical parts of the history taking.
- *Examine*: Document any unusual bruises, burns or scratches that you find. Note their locations, shapes and colours. Abdomens and inner thighs are not common places for accidental bruises.

Obstetrics

Domestic abuse is a major cause of maternal and foetal death. You must ask every pregnant woman about domestic abuse; do not make the mistake of thinking that someone else (e.g. the midwife or GP) will have asked. You can cross domestic abuse off your list of concerns only by asking yourself (see Box 16.2).

Box 16.2 Factors that should raise suspicion of domestic violence in pregnancy

- Patient books late or does not attend clinics.
- Patient repeatedly presents with minor problems or repeat admissions.
- Patient self-discharges or does not complete treatments.
- Patient is persistently depressed, anxious or self-harming.
- Patient has injuries, especially on the abdomen, breasts, inner thighs, head and neck, and makes light of them.
- Patient experiences frequent vaginal discharge, postcoital bleeding, urine infection or pelvic pain.
- Patient experiences recurrent miscarriages, unexplained stillbirths or preterm labour.
- There is intrauterine growth restriction or low birth weight.
- Pregnancy is unplanned or unwanted.
- Patient makes a termination request or has undergone multiple terminations.
- Patient is unable to stop smoking or there is other substance misuse.

Box 16.2 lists factors to look out for in pregnant women, gleaned from the Confidential Enquiry into Maternal Deaths (Lewis *et al.*, 2004). Many of these factors apply in any consultation, not just obstetrics.

Women who experience domestic or sexual violence are more likely to have an obstetric complication that can threaten their lives directly, as well as indirectly if they are prevented from attending antenatal care. They are more likely to have:

- Premature labour.
- Chorioamnionitis.
- Antepartum haemorrhage.

- Stillbirth.
- Low-birth weight baby.

They are also more likely to request a caesarean section for nonobstetric reasons.

Such women should be considered high-risk pregnancies and require more than standard antenatal care.

If a patient has been subjected to female genital mutilation, this can necessitate corrective reversal surgery before she can deliver vaginally and there will be midwifery child safeguarding issues (see Chapter 17).

Gynaecology

Women suffering domestic or sexual violence are at increased risk of gynaecological problems, such as:

- Menstrual disorders (menorrhagia or dysmenorrhoea).
- Pelvic pain.
- Dyspareunia.
- Vaginal discharge.
- Pelvic inflammatory disease.
- Postcoital bleeding.
- Failure to attend for cervical smears.

Gynaecologists have recently seen a rise in requests for cosmetic labial surgery. In some cases, such patients are experiencing 'pudendal disgust' following sexual assault or humiliating comments. They may be being pressured by a controlling partner into having disfiguring surgery in order to attain a style seen only in airbrushed pornography. Such requests must always be considered in the context of possible abuse and low self-esteem.

Contraception

Abused women are more likely to have an unintended pregnancy. They may subsequently be forced to have a termination by their partner or they may themselves opt to not have a child in the context of a violent relationship but be terrified that the partner will find out and become more violent or force them to continue with the pregnancy.

An abusive, controlling partner will try to control contraception, so women may be better off with an implant or intrauterine contraceptive device (IUCD; see Box 16.3) than oral contraception as these are harder for the partner to stop. Depot-Provera injections are another possible method, provided that the woman can attend regularly. A patient may repeatedly attend for emergency contraception in an attempt to control her fertility.

Box 16.3 Long-acting reversible contraception (LARC)

- Contraceptive implant, e.g. Implanon/Nexplanon.
- Contraceptive injection, e.g. Depot-Provera.
- IUCD, e.g. T cu 389s.
- Intrauterine system (IUS), e.g. Mirena.

It has been shown that women who are victims of abuse are more likely to request sterilisation. As this is a more invasive procedure than LARC, consider why a patient is requesting sterilisation:

- Is it in the context of a relationship where the partner is demanding it?
- Is it because it is the only way she will be in control of her contraception?
- Is it because the partner has convinced her she is a lousy mother?
- Is it that she or her partner is unaware of the other methods?

Genitourinary medicine

A woman experiencing domestic or sexual violence may present to genitourinary medicine due to:

- Vaginal discharge.
- Catching a sexually transmitted disease (STD) from her partner.
- Being forced to have sex with others for her partner's financial gain.
- Being raped by her partner.

If a woman has been raped, she may not want to go to the police. She may think, wrongly, that they would not take it seriously. She may still be worried that she has been harmed and that this will affect her future childbearing.

Remember that young adolescents may also be in abusive relationships; this is not a problem that only affects the over-20s. Also, a significant proportion of sex workers have had adverse experiences in childhood, including abuse and living in care. They too face continuing risks of abuse, violence and STDs.

Women with HIV may have experienced various forms of gender-based violence over many years and in different countries (see Box 16.4). Women living with HIV have to manage complex health and personal issues, which often include abuse. An inner-London study of women living with HIV (largely black African) found that over half had experienced intimate partner violence at some point in their lives. Women with HIV are often diagnosed as the result of antenatal HIV testing, when they may face many conflicting priorities. Their needs are complex and can involve a range of medical, legal, social and voluntary services.

Box 16.4 Gender-based violence and the links with HIV

The definition of violence against HIV-positive women is any act, structure or process in which power is exerted in such a way as to cause physical, sexual, psychological, financial or legal harm.

- For migrant women, gender-based violence in all its forms may have taken place in their home country or en route to the UK. In addition, it may be ongoing in the UK.

- The woman may have acquired HIV through rape.
- Rape is extremely common in some countries with high HIV prevalence, such as South Africa, and in conflict zones.
- Women can be the victims of trafficking and forced transactional sex for money, housing and food.
- Domestic violence can be exacerbated by male disempowerment related to differences in the status of women in the UK compared with the home country.
- HIV status can be used by partners or acquaintances to establish both financial and emotional power within relationships.
- Partners may make threats to abandon the family and to disclose serostatus to friends, family and coworkers (in some cases via social media Web sites).
- Partners may threaten disclosure to social services, claiming that their children will be removed.
- Women with HIV may fear prosecution for reckless transmission.
- Institutional abuse includes refusal by nurses to treat HIV-positive women and poor practice within statutory housing services that fail to understand discrimination perpetrated against female clients living with HIV.
- Women and their children may be dependent on their abusers emotionally, financially and socially, e.g. for:
  - Food and housing (and lack of recourse to public funds may make it difficult to leave the abuser).
  - Health care and travel to reach it.
  - Language skills (to help negotiate support).
  - Access to their cultural and religious community.

Further reading

Dalton, M. (2013) *Forensic Gynaecology*. RCOG Press, London.

Dalton, M. (2013) *Best Practice & Research: Clinical Obstetrics & Gynaecology*, Volume 27, Issue 1. Elsevier.

Dhairyawan, R., Tariq, S., Scourse, R. & Coyne, K. (2012) Intimate partner violence in women living with HIV attending an inner city clinic in the UK: prevalence and associated factors. Poster presentation at BHIVA 2012.

Lewis, G., Drife, J., Clutton-Brock, T., Cooper, G., Hall, M., Harper, A., Hepburn, M., Neilson, J., Nelson-Piercy, C., McClure, J., Oates, M., Penney, G., Sallah, K., de Swiet, M., Millward-Sadler, H., Vlies, R., Brace, V., Dattani, N., Macfarlane, A., Physick, N., Ronsmans, C., Hunt, L., Chamberlain, J. & Corbin, T. (2004) Why Mothers Die 2000–2002: The Sixth Report of the Confidential Enquiries into Maternal Deaths in the United Kingdom, http://www.hqip.org.uk/assets/NCAPOP-Library/CMACE-Reports/33.-2004-Why-Mothers-Die-2000-2002-The-Sixth-Report-of-the-Confidential-Enquiries-into-Maternal-Deaths-in-the-UK.pdf (last accessed 12 February 2014).

The Sophia Forum (2013) *HIV as a Cause or Consequence of HIV for Women in England: A Feasibility Study Regarding a Potential National Investigation*, http://www.sophiaforum.net/resources/Finalweb_SophiaForum_HIV_GBVreport2013.pdf (last accessed 12 February 2014).

Royal College of Obstetrics and Gynaecology (no date) ATSM: forensic gynaecology, http://www.rcog.org.uk/curriculum-module/atsm-forensic-gynaecology (last accessed 12 February 2014).

CHAPTER 17

Female Genital Mutilation

Sarah M. Creighton

Department of Women's Health, University College London Hospital, UK

OVERVIEW

- Female genital mutilation (FGM) or female circumcision is a deeply rooted tradition
- FGM is practised by specific ethnic groups in Africa, Asia and the Middle East
- It consists of various procedures that remove or damage the external female genital organs
- There is no medical reason for FGM and it has no health benefits
- It is often performed in unsterile conditions and without pain relief
- It causes severe short- and long-term damage to both physical and psychological health

---

What is FGM?

FGM is defined by the World Health Organization (WHO) as a set of procedures that intentionally alter or cause injury to the female genital organs for nonmedical reasons. It is almost always carried out on children and is recognised as a violation of the human rights of girls and women. It also constitutes an extreme form of discrimination against women and a violation of the rights of children.

It is estimated that 140 million girls and women are living with the consequences of FGM and that a further 3 million girls undergo FGM in Africa each year. It is now recognised that FGM also occurs outside Africa, in some countries in Asia and the Middle East. FGM is increasingly identified in the UK amongst migrants from FGM-practising countries.

Why is FGM performed?

Various explanations are given and these vary within countries and communities. However, the single underlying and unifying reason is the control of sexuality in women. Individual communities may cite the following reasons:

- Social pressure.
- The necessary preparation of a girl for adulthood and marriage.

- A cultural ideal of modesty to remove 'unclean' body parts.
- The need reduce female libido and ensure chastity.
- Religious beliefs (although no religious scripts recommend FGM).
- Cementing or maintenance of cultural identity.

What does FGM consist of?

FGM is usually performed by traditional circumcisers. However, the WHO estimates that 18% of all FGM is performed by health care providers. This percentage may be increasing.

The WHO has classified FGM into four major types:

1 *Clitoridectomy*: Partial or total removal of the clitoris, or in rare cases only the prepuce (skin over the clitoris).
2 *Excision*: Partial or total removal of the clitoris and labia minora, with or without removal or the labia majora.
3 *Infibulation*: Narrowing of the vaginal opening through the creation of a covering seal. The seal is formed by cutting and repositioning the labia minora or majora with or without removal of the clitoris.
4 *Other*: All other harmful procedures to the genitals for non-medical reasons, e.g. pricking, piercing, incision, scraping and cauterising.

The procedure is performed without anaesthetic and in the absence of sterile conditions. The child is usually forcibly restrained while the external genitalia are removed using a knife, scalpel or other sharp tool, such as a razor blade or piece of glass. The wound is then covered with herbal paste and the legs are bound. If the vagina has been closed, a straw or reed is placed inside it to allow it to heal over, leaving a small opening for later micturition and menstruation.

Outcomes

There are no health benefits to FGM. The risks are given in Table 17.1.

Legal status in the UK

It has been illegal to perform FGM in the UK since 1985. In 2003 the law was extended to make it illegal to take a girl out of the

ABC of Domestic and Sexual Violence, First Edition.
Edited by Susan Bewley and Jan Welch.
© 2014 John Wiley & Sons, Ltd. Published 2014 by John Wiley & Sons, Ltd.

Table 17.1 Risks of FGM.

Immediate/short term	Long term
Death	Recurrent urinary infections
Pain	Keloid scarring and cysts
Shock	Painful menstruation
Tetanus and gangrene	Infertility
Sepsis	Dyspareunia
Haemorrhage	Psychosexual and psychological difficulties
Urinary retention	The need for further surgery to the
Damage to urethra and anus	vagina to allow intercourse and vaginal birth
Bloodborne infections, e.g. HIV, hepatitis B and C	Increased obstetric complications, including postpartum haemorrhage, perineal trauma and perinatal death

UK for FGM. Perpetrators face a large fine and up to 15 years in prison. Anecdotal stories suggest that FGM is currently available in the UK, but to date there have been no successful prosecutions. 'Cutters' may be flown in by families and communities or a 'holiday' for the child or teenager may be arranged. It has been suggested that 66 000 women in the UK have had FGM, with a further 20 000 girls at risk. These figures are out of date and are very likely to be an underestimate.

Management of FGM in the UK

There are two aspects to FGM management: provision of sensitive and appropriate services to women who have undergone FGM and safeguarding of girls at risk of FGM.

Provision of services

Some hospitals in high-prevalence areas have specialist FGM clinics. The commonest reason for referral is for deinfibulation. Deinfibulation is a procedure that divides the scar tissue covering the vagina in women with type 3 FGM. It may be required to allow sexual intercourse. If a woman is pregnant, deinfibulation may be required to open the lower vagina and facilitate delivery of the baby. Deinfibulation is often called a 'reversal' of FGM, although it does not replace any of the sensitive genital tissues that have been removed. It is usually performed under local anaesthetic in the outpatient clinic, although on occasion a day-case admission and general or spinal anaesthetic may be required. Psychological and psychosexual concerns may also need addressing, although many clinics do not offer access to such specialised services.

Safeguarding

The main risk factor for FGM is to be born into an FGM-practising community. All pregnant women will have some contact with health care services and this is an ideal opportunity for safeguarding. All pregnant women should be asked about FGM and those that have undergone FGM should be informed about its health risks and its legal status in the UK. The fact that the mother has had FGM should be documented in the infant's red book and this information must be passed on to the GP and health visitor. Existing girls in the family may also be at risk. It is recognised that health care professionals find these questions difficult to address. If there is a suspicion that a child is at risk of FGM, health care professionals should contact their local safeguarding team. Outside health care settings, the police or children's social services can be contacted, and the Foreign Office runs a non-urgent helpline.

Medicalisation

In many countries, doctors offer FGM procedures – often for money – in place of traditional circumcisers. This is widely condemned by international medical organisations. Although deinfibulation can be offered to women, particularly before childbirth, there is no good evidence for complex so-called 'reconstructive surgery' in terms of sexual function and complications.

Conclusion

FGM offers no health benefits and carries severe short- and long-term risks. Women who have undergone FGM will require specialised care during pregnancy and delivery. Girls born within FGM-practising communities are at risk of FGM both abroad and in the UK. It is essential that health care professionals remain vigilant about FGM and are aware of the appropriate steps to take when they suspect a child is at risk.

Further reading

HM Government (no date) *Multi-Agency Practice Guidelines: Female Genital Mutilation*, http://www.openeyecommunications.com/wp-content/uploads/2011/02/FGM.pdf (last accessed 12 February 2014).

Royal College of Obstetricians and Gynaecologists (2009) Female genital mutilation and its management, http://www.rcog.org.uk/files/rcog-corp/GreenTop53FemaleGenitalMutilation.pdf (last accessed 12 February 2014).

"Tackling FGM in the UK. Intercollegiate recommendations for identifying, recording and reporting". 12 February 2014. Published by The Royal College of Midwives.

World Health Organization (2000) Female genital mutilation, http://www.who.int/mediacentre/factsheets/fs241/en/ (last accessed 12 February 2014).

Web sites

FGM National Clinic Group, www.fgmnationalgroup.org (last accessed 12 February 2014).

Forward, www.forwarduk.org (last accessed 12 February 2014).

CHAPTER 18

Sexual Violence: What to Consider First

Catherine White

Sexual Assault Referral Centre, St Mary's Manchester, UK

OVERVIEW

- Sexual assault is common but hard for victims to disclose
- Physical and psychological consequences can be severe and long-lasting
- Offering choices can help victims regain control lost through the assault
- Immediate considerations include safety and medical, forensic and psychological needs

---

Disclosure of sexual assault

Victims of sexual violence may present in a number of ways (Box 18.1), some obvious but others easily overlooked. Remember it may be incredibly difficult for victims to talk about what has happened to them.

Box 18.1 **Some ways a sexual assault or rape victim might present**

- Direct disclosure of assault (acute or historic).
- Request for emergency contraception.
- Sexually transmitted infection (STI) screening.
- HIV post-exposure prophylaxis.
- Unwanted pregnancy.
- Victim of physical violence, including domestic violence.
- Depression, anxiety, psychosis, chronic pelvic pain, dyspareunia, drug and alcohol misuse, self-harm and suicide.

Sexual violence and abuse can cause severe, long-lasting harm to individuals in a range of ways: health, social and economic. It can worsen inequalities, which mostly affect women, the vulnerable and the disadvantaged, and is often linked to domestic violence – see Box 18.2.

ABC of Domestic and Sexual Violence, First Edition.
Edited by Susan Bewley and Jan Welch.
© 2014 John Wiley & Sons, Ltd. Published 2014 by John Wiley & Sons, Ltd.

Box 18.2 **Statistics re sexual violence**

- 1 in 4 women have been abused during their lifetime.
- 1 in 5 girls and 1 in 10 boys experience some form of childhood sexual abuse.
- 1 in 40 adult women and 1 in 200 adult men (aged 16–59) were sexually assaulted in 2010–11 in the UK.
- 3.1 million women have been sexually assaulted since the age of 16.
- 40–50% of women experiencing physically abusive domestic violence are also raped.
- 70% of female mental health inpatients have experienced physical or sexual abuse.
- Just under 50% of female mental health service users have been subjected to sexual abuse.
- Around 50% of female mental health service users have been subjected to physical abuse in childhood, notwithstanding adult abuse, which they may also experience.
- 23% of women and 3% of men experience sexual assault as an adult.

Offering choices and options

Sexual violence is about control. During the assault, the victim has no control over what happens to them. An important element of aiding recovery is to offer back control as soon as possible.

Your task is to:

- Assess what a person might need.
- Explain this to them in a way that they can understand.
- Offer them choices.

You will need to have an idea of what is entailed (Table 18.1), the timescales involved and who your relevant local service providers are (e.g. a local sexual assault referral centre, SARC).

Consent and confidentiality

From the outset, before information is divulged, the clinician must make the limitations of confidentiality very clear to the patient.

If the case proceeds along the criminal justice route then it is highly likely that there will be a request for the medical notes to be disclosed to the courts.

Table 18.1 Things to consider when someone discloses rape.

Immediate safety	• Are they safe? • Are there any children or other dependents to consider? • Are any safeguarding referrals required? • Are you safe?
Medical needs	• Injuries, assessment and treatment • Emergency contraception • HIV post-exposure prophylaxis following sexual exposure (PEPSE) • Hepatitis B PEPSE • Screening for sexually transmitted infections • Pregnancy testing
Forensic needs	• Preservation of evidence • Documentation of injuries, including photography where necessary • Documentation of allegations • All to a standard so that evidence is admissible in court
Psychological needs	• Of the complainant (including risk of self-harm, suicide) • Of other witnesses • Of yourself and other members of staff

Equally, the patient must be aware that should information be divulged which suggests that children or vulnerable adults are at risk then it will be necessary to share this information.

When does a patient's disclosure put a doctor under a duty to report to someone else, such as social services or the police?

Whether victims want to report the abuse to police or social services or not, the doctor must weigh their wishes against the doctor's duty to protect them and also any possible threat to others posed by the alleged offender.

In the UK, you would always report to police, social care and safeguarding teams:

• Child victims who are not Gillick-competent.
• Adult victims with a permanent loss of capacity.

If unsure, you can consult a variety of sources, including senior colleagues, safeguarding teams, local child protection guidelines, medical defence organisation and so on. The UK Faculty of Forensic and Legal Medicine (FFLM) has produced guidelines for clinicians dealing with a patient who may have been assaulted and seems not to have full capacity (Faculty of Forensic and Legal Medicine, 2011).

Remember that gaining consent from any patient is always important (Box 18.3). This is especially relevant with the sexual assault victim, who has had power and control taken from them during the assault.

Box 18.3 **Remember the key elements of consent**

For consent to be valid, it must be given *voluntarily* by an appropriately *informed* person (the patient, or where relevant someone with parental responsibility for a patient under the age of 18) who has the *capacity* to consent to the intervention in question.

Acquiescence where the person does not know what the intervention entails is not 'consent'.

Capacity and the Mental Capacity Act

The definition of, assessment of and responsibilities in relation to capacity (also known as mental capacity) in England and Wales are laid out in the Mental Capacity Act (MCA) 2005.

The MCA applies to all adults aged 16 and over. It defines 'capacity' as the ability to make a decision (see Box 18.4). It relates to the *process* of making a decision and not to the *outcome* of the decision. It is not limited to medical decisions but can apply to any decision-making process.

Box 18.4 **The key issues of capacity**

• All adults are *presumed to have capacity* unless there is evidence to the contrary.
• Capacity is *task specific*. A person may be capable of deciding one issue but not another.
• Capacity is also *time specific*. A person's capacity may alter with time.

The MCA defines lack of capacity thus: if, at the time the decision needs to be made, a patient is unable to make the decision because of an 'impairment of, or a disturbance in the functioning of, the mind or brain', they are deemed incapable.

The term 'capacity' was previously used interchangeably with the term 'competence'. Since the MCA 2005, 'capacity' is the preferred term.

The MCA lays out five statutory principles

• A person must be assumed to have capacity unless it is established otherwise.
• A person is not to be treated as unable to make a decision unless all practicable steps to help him or her to do so have failed. (Note that this includes communicating in an appropriate way; the clinician may need to arrange for interpreters or signers to be present or use visual aids.)
• A person is not to be treated as unable to make a decision merely because he or she makes an unwise decision.
• An action or a decision taken under this Act for or on behalf of a person who lacks capacity must be taken in his or her best interests.
• Before the action or decision is taken, consider whether its purpose can be as effectively achieved in a way that is less restrictive of the person's rights and freedom of action.

Health care professionals are warned that a person cannot be judged to lack capacity simply because of age, appearance or behaviour.

Assessment of capacity

In order to assess someone's capacity to make a valid treatment decision, consider two criteria:

1 Do they have an impairment of mind or brain (temporary or permanent)?
2 Does the impairment mean that the person is unable to make the decision in question, at the time at which it needs to be made (see Box 18.5)?

Box 18.5 **Determining whether someone is able to make a decision**

Is the person in question:

- Able to understand what the decision is?
- Capable of choosing and able to understand why a choice is needed?
- Informed about risks, benefits and alternatives?
- Retaining and understanding enough basic information to make a choice?
- Aware of how the decision is relevant to him/herself?
- Aware that there is a right to consent or refuse?
- Able to refuse?
- Capable of communicating a choice?

The issues to consider when dealing with an alleged or suspected assault on a person with reduced capacity are shown in Figure 18.1.

Time frames that matter

Always assess and manage life-threatening medical issues first (Table 18.2).

History taking

History taking needs to be:

- Accurate.
- Contemporaneous.
- Comprehensive.
- Objective.
- Respectful and sensitive.
- Paced at the patient's rate, not the clinician's.
- Intelligent and tailored to the circumstances and the findings.

Any notes made should:

- Be legible.
- Clearly state who made them.
- Clearly state who gave information and who was present when it was given.
- Be signed and dated.
- Be stored safely.

See also chapter 20.

Pro formas are available (e.g. from www.fflm.ac.uk) to act as an aide-memoire.

The examination

- Should ideally be done by someone who specialises in sexual assault examinations.
- Should be performed in an age-appropriate, forensically sound (contamination-free) environment.
- Privacy must be ensured.
- Should be explained as you go along.
- Should go at the victim's pace.
- Contemporaneous notes must be made.
- All negative as well as positive findings must be recorded.
- Should include height, weight, mental state, review of systems, information on clothing, signs of intoxication etc.

A forensic examination should include inspection of all body surfaces and not just the genitalia. Research shows that a person is more likely to sustain injuries on general body surfaces rather than the genitalia (see Table 18.3 and Box 18.6).

Box 18.6 **Features to record when documenting injuries**

- Type of injury.
- Size.
- Shape.
- Depth (if possible, e.g. laceration).
- Edges (e.g. abraded, healing).
- Colour.
- Surface covering (scab formation, crusting).
- Swelling.
- Tenderness.
- Distance from fixed anatomical site.
- Explanation, if offered (noted verbatim).

Do always consider the differential diagnosis of any findings. Particularly in children, some medical conditions can mimic injury, such as Lichen sclerosus et atrophicus or Mongolian blue spots.

Forensic samples

Locard's principle

Dr Edmond Locard (1877–1966), the 'French Sherlock Holmes', coined the phrase 'every contact leaves a trace' (see Figure 18.2). Bearing this in mind, what samples are taken will depend upon factors such as the nature of the assault, the time since it occurred and any subsequent actions taken (see Faculty of Forensic and Legal Medicine, 2011).

If the victim is being transferred elsewhere for the forensic examination or there is likely to be any significant delay, consider the use of early evidence kits to preserve evidence (see Chapter 12, Figure 12.1).

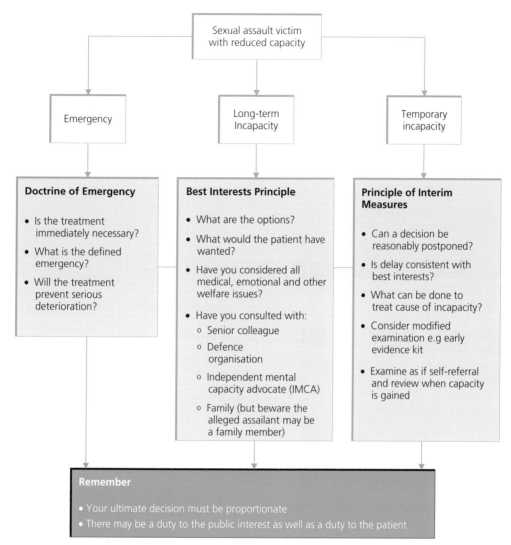

Figure 18.1 Alleged or suspected sexual assault on a person with reduced capacity: issues the forensic physician must consider. IMCA, independent mental capacity advocate.

Table 18.2 Timing issues when dealing with sexual assault (see also Chapter 19).

Issue	Action	Time frame
Emergency contraception	Levonelle	A single oral dose of 3 mg as soon as possible after unprotected sex and within 72 hours
	Ulipristal	One 30 mg tablet, orally, as soon as possible, but no later than 120 hours after unprotected sexual intercourse
	Copper intrauterine contraceptive device	Up to 5 days after ovulation
Post-exposure prophylaxis following sexual exposure (PEPSE)	HIV	As soon as possible within 72 hours
	Hepatitis B	Up to 6 weeks
Forensic samples	Mouth	2 days
Take *as soon as possible*	Female genitalia	7 days (12 hours if digital vaginal penetration)
Check www.fflm.ac.uk for latest updates	Male genitalia	3 days
Different time frames apply to some samples for prepubertal children	Anal swabs	3 days (12 hours if digital anal penetration)
	Urine for toxicology	3 days (14 days if drug-facilitated sexual assault suspected)
Times shown here are maximum rather than expected persistence	Blood for toxicology	3 days
	Skin	7 days
Injuries	Most rape victims will have no or very few injuries.	
	Some of the injuries that can be very significant forensically may be very minor in nature and heal rapidly, i.e. within days.	
Safety	Assessment of personal safety of victim and relevant third parties	Immediate

Table 18.3 Injuries.

Bruises

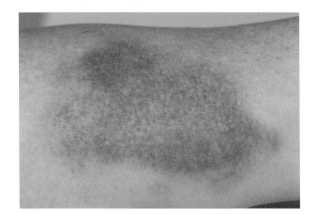

Caused by blunt force
May not appear immediately
Under force of gravity may appear at a site distant from the site of original trauma
Difficult to age
Also called ecchymoses, contusion, haematoma

Abrasion

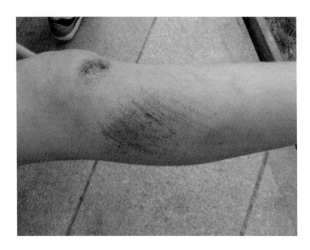

Superficial disruption of surface epithelium
May bleed
Do not extend or gravitate
Also called by nonmedical terms such as 'graze' or 'scratch'
Signs of healing should be documented, e.g. fresh bleeding, scab formation

Laceration

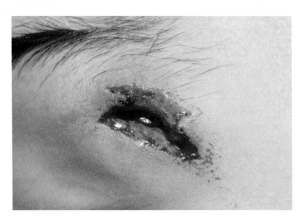

Full-thickness split of the skin caused by blunt trauma
Irregular edges and irregular division of tissue planes
Tissue bridges, including blood vessels and nerves, may be visible
May have abraded bruised margin
May contain debris
Often bleed

(continued overleaf)

Table 18.3 *(continued)*

Incision

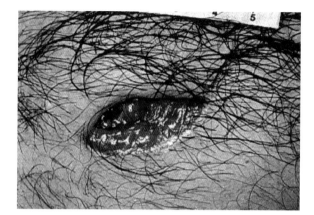

Caused by sharp objects breaching the epithelium

Sometimes known as 'cuts'

Edges tend to be straight, with no associated bruising or abrasion

Tissues are cut in the same plane, with nerves and blood vessels cleanly divided

May bleed profusely

Burn

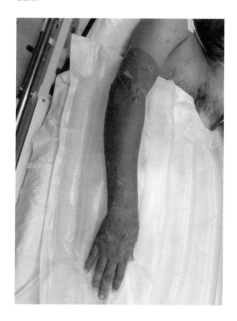

Can be caused by heat or chemical sources

Can be caused deliberately by cigarettes

Bite

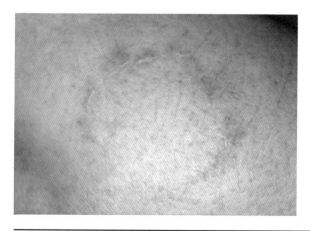

May contain a mixture of bruises, abrasions or lacerations

It is important to take swabs for saliva

Photographs, if correctly taken, can be used to help identify the assailant

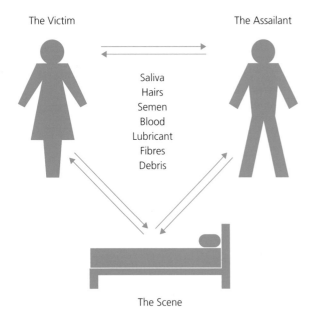

The Victim   The Assailant

Saliva
Hairs
Semen
Blood
Lubricant
Fibres
Debris

The Scene

Figure 18.2 Locard's principle. Source: White 2010. Adapted with permission from Dr Catherine White and St Mary's Hospital, Manchester.

Chain of custody

For forensic evidence to be admissible in a criminal justice process, there must be a 'chain of custody', clearly documenting:

- Where the samples came from.
- Who took the samples.
- Who has had possession of the samples since they were taken, and when.
- How the samples have been stored and looked after since they were taken.

Male rape

Men and boys are also victims of sexual violence. It may be that it is even more of a taboo subject for men and that it is harder for them to disclose than it is for women (see Chapter 6).

Summary

Table 18.4 provides some tips for good clinical practice, while case studies are given in Boxes 18.7 and 18.8.

Box 18.7 **Case study**

Georgina Green is a 20-year-old law student. She presents to A&E on a Sunday morning asking for 'the morning-after pill'. She seems distracted and upset. *What should you do?*

- **Option A**: Prescribe progesterone-only emergency contraception and discharge her.
- **Option B**: Explore why she is asking for the morning-after pill. Be alert to nonverbal cues that might raise suspicions and thereby give her the opportunity to disclose more information to you.

If you chose Option A, go back to the beginning and read the chapter again. If you chose Option B, well done! Now read on …

Georgina says that at a party last night she bumped into her ex-boyfriend. 'Although I said "no", he forced me to have sex.' (That is, it appears to be rape.) *What should you do?*

- **Option A**: Phone the police immediately.
- **Option B**: Discuss with Georgina what she would like to do and what her options are. Consider the forensic, medical, psychological and any safeguarding aspects. If unsure, seek advice from someone who can help, such as a local SARC.

If you chose Option A, go back to the beginning and read the chapter again. If you chose Option B, well done!

Box 18.8 **Case study**

Mo Mainwaring is a 77–year-old retired bank manager. He was living alone until his stroke last year. His 50-year-old son moved in to care for him. Mo's speech has been difficult to understand since the stroke. He seems to have become quite withdrawn in mood. Today he presents with 'bleeding down below' and on examination you notice a few anal fissures. *What should you do?*

- **Option A**: Advise Mo that he is probably constipated due to his lack of mobility and prescribe some lactulose.
- **Option B**: Take time to ask about his general health and well being. Give him some privacy and explore what might be going on for him.

If you chose Option A, go back to the beginning and read the chapter again. If you chose Option B, well done! Now read on …

Mo gets very upset and gradually discloses that his son gets frustrated and hits him. Sometimes, when drunk, his son sexually assaults him. Mo is frightened of going back home but does not want to get his son into trouble. *What should you do?*

- **Option A**: Arrange for the district nurses to go in and help with Mo's care on a regular basis, thereby taking some of the pressure off the son.
- **Option B**: Assess Mo's immediate forensic and health needs. Assume he has capacity (unless there is evidence to the contrary) and let him make informed decisions. Consider his immediate safety, including a safeguarding referral. Seek help from senior colleagues.

If you chose Option A, go back to the beginning and read the chapter again. If you chose Option B, well done!

Further reading

Department of Health (2003) Mainstreaming gender and women's mental health: implementation guidance, http://webarchive.nationalarchives.gov.uk/20130107105354/http://www.dh.gov.uk/en/Publicationsandstatistics/Publications/PublicationsPolicyAndGuidance/DH_4072067 (last accessed 12 February 2014).

Table 18.4 Good clinician practice and the victim of sexual violence.

Do	Don't
Consider the possibility of sexual violence as the reason for a patient presenting	Panic
Treat with respect and sensitivity	Be judgemental and disbelieving
Offer informed realistic choices	Be paternalistic
Consider medical, psychological and forensic needs	Take signs and symptoms at face value
Be prepared with information on local services	Be clueless as to local services
Seek advice from more experienced clinicians	Struggle on your own
Make careful comprehensive contemporaneous notes	Jot down a few miserable lines. This will not help you remember the details you need when giving evidence in court months later
Use body maps for injuries	Run the risk of letting someone down
Consider safeguarding issues for the victim and third parties	Expect to be unaffected by what you have heard and seen
Look after yourself – these cases can be upsetting	

Department of Health (2008) Refocusing the Care Programme Approach: policy and positive practice guidance, http://webarchive.nationalarchives.gov.uk/20130107105354/http://www.dh.gov.uk/en/Publicationsandstatistics/Publications/PublicationsPolicyAndGuidance/DH_083647 (last accessed 12 February 2014).

Faculty of Forensic and Legal Medicine (2011) Consent from patients who may have been physically assaulted, http://fflm.ac.uk/upload/documents/1311675189.pdf (last accessed 12 February 2014).

Flatley, J., Kershaw, C., Smith, K., Chaplin, R. & Moon, D. (2010) Crime in England and Wales 2009/10: findings from the British Crime Survey and police recorded crime, https://www.gov.uk/government/uploads/system/uploads/attachment_data/file/116347/hosb1210.pdf (last accessed 12 February 2014).

General Medical Council (2009) *Confidentiality*, http://www.gmc-uk.org/guidance/ethical_guidance/confidentiality.asp (last accessed 12 February 2014).

HM Government (2011) Crime in England and Wales 2010 to 2011, http://www.homeoffice.gov.uk/publications/science-research-statistics/research-statistics/crime-research/hosb1011/ (last accessed 12 February 2014).

Martin, E.K., Taft, C.T. & Resick, P.A. (2007) A review of marital rape. *Aggression and Violent Behavior*, **12**(3), 329–347.

Smith, K., Osborne, S., Lau, I. & Britton, A. (2012) Homicides, Firearm Offences and Intimate Violence 2010/11: Supplementary Volume 2 to Crime in England and Wales 2010/11, https://www.gov.uk/government/uploads/system/uploads/attachment_data/file/116483/hosb0212.pdf (last accessed 12 February 2014).

White, C. (2010) *Sexual Assault, A Forensic Physician's Practice Guide*. St Mary's Centre.

CHAPTER 19

Rape and Sexual Assault: Medical and Psychosocial Care

Hannah Loftus and Karen Rogstad

Genitourinary Medicine, Sheffield Teaching Hospitals NHS Foundation Trust, UK

OVERVIEW

- Individuals presenting following sexual assault are vulnerable. Medical and psychosocial care must be correct first time

- The consultation and examination should be carried out at the victim's pace and tailored to their needs

- Victims of rape and sexual assault should be offered testing for sexually transmitted infections (STIs) and consideration should be given to post-exposure prophylaxis

- STI samples might be used as evidence in a court of law and should thus have a chain of evidence

- All women and girls should be assessed for, and have access to, emergency contraception, including those who are pubertal and perimenopausal

- Psychosocial support should be available both immediately and in the long term

---

Introduction

The medical care of individuals presenting following sexual assault needs to be managed sensitively but with awareness of relevant time considerations. Most people who have been sexually assaulted do seek medical help at some stage, but the time taken to do so may range from hours to years. Management will vary depending on the time since the assault, whether the individual chooses to report the assault to the police and where she or he chooses to receive after-care. Immediate care (see Chapter 18) should be followed up with longer-term medical and psychosocial support.

If there are ongoing potentially life-threatening problems, their management takes precedence and the patient should be transferred to an emergency department immediately.

The individual should be asked if they wish to report to the police. If they do then transfer to a sexual assault referral centre (SARC) should be facilitated. Even if they do not wish to report, a SARC provides the ideal environment for assessment and support. However, some patients may choose not to access these services.

Accurate and legible documentation in the notes is extremely important; records should be timed and dated (see Chapter 20). The notes may be used as evidence if the patient chooses to report the assault to the police at a later time. Detailed documentation can also be invaluable later for other reasons, such as an application to the Criminal Injuries Compensation Authority. In all departments where individuals commonly present following sexual assault, a pro forma can be useful in enabling inexperienced staff to collect all necessary information.

History

The history should be carried out in a private room where the patient can feel safe. They should be given time to talk and should never be pressured into giving information they do not wish to disclose. It is important to ask about details of the sexual assault if these have not already been given or are unavailable. This helps in determining risk, tailoring testing and treatment and providing appropriate support. Specific details concerning the assault and the perpetrator will help to identify the need for STI screening, pregnancy prevention, psychosocial support or a forensic medical examination. The patient should also be asked whether they have any injuries.

A sexual history should be taken, including current contraceptive use and date of last menstrual period, as well as last consensual intercourse. A full medical history is important and should include previous illnesses, including mental health. A full medication history should include use of asthma inhalers and alternative therapies, which are relevant if post-exposure prophylaxis for HIV is given. It is also important to determine to whom the victim has disclosed the assault. Information should not normally be passed on without their consent.

Examination and tests

It is good practice to offer a full examination, but this may be a reminder of the assault. Self-taken or noninvasive tests for STIs may be offered as an alternative. Both men and women should be offered proctoscopy if there is a history of anal penetration.

Early evidence kits (see Chapters 12 and 18) are used by police to allow early collection of DNA evidence and toxicology. These kits generally include a urine sample pot, mouth swab and mouth

---

ABC of Domestic and Sexual Violence, First Edition.
Edited by Susan Bewley and Jan Welch.

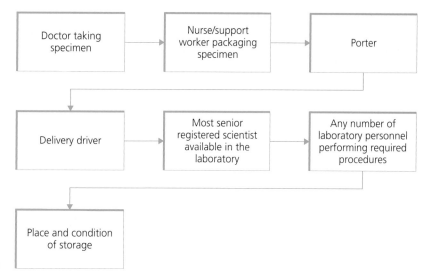

Figure 19.1 Who may be involved in a chain of evidence.

rinse. They can be offered in a non-SARC setting if the patient wishes to report at a later date or to allow sharing of information on an anonymous basis. A chain of evidence form should ideally be used for all specimens taken, which will involve several individuals (Figure 19.1). All police and SARC services have procedures in place for chain of evidence but it is also possible to put them in place in sexual health services, for both forensic and microbiological samples.

Prevention of pregnancy

There is a 5% risk of pregnancy in women of reproductive age following rape. Prevention of pregnancy must be a primary consideration when a woman presents following a sexual assault. Pregnancy testing should be considered prior to the offer of emergency contraception. Note that a negative pregnancy test does not reliably exclude pregnancy if there has been unprotected sexual intercourse in the preceding 3 weeks.

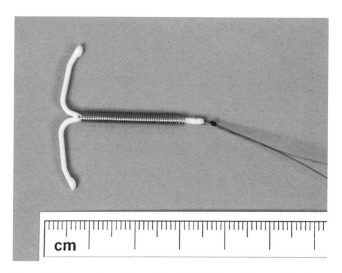

Figure 19.2 Copper intrauterine device (CuIUD). Source: Rogstad (2011). Reproduced by permission of John Wiley & Sons, Ltd.

A copper intrauterine device (CuIUD) is the most effective form of emergency contraception (see Box 19.1 and Figure 19.2). For those women who decline a CuIUD, hormonal methods should be offered (Box 19.2).

Box 19.1 **Emergency contraception: copper intrauterine device (CuIUD)**

This option should be discussed with all women who present within the 'window of opportunity'.

- If the assault was less than 5 days (120 hours) ago and there have been no other episodes of unprotected sexual intercourse since the last menstrual period, a CuIUD can be fitted at any point in the menstrual cycle.
- If the assault was more than 5 days ago, or if there have been two or more episodes of unprotected sexual intercourse since the last menstrual period, a CuIUD can be fitted up to 5 days after the earliest expected date of ovulation (i.e. day 19 of a 28 day cycle, which is 5 days after presumed ovulation).

A CuIUD can be fitted in a nulliparous women.
The CuIUD can be removed any time after pregnancy has been excluded (e.g. at onset of menstrual period).
If a client presents to a service where CuIUDs are not fitted, a timely referral pathway should be put in place and consideration should be given to providing oral emergency contraception in the meantime.

Box 19.2 **Emergency contraception: hormonal methods**

Levonorgestrel

- Levonelle 1500® (levonorgestrel) is licensed for use up to 72 hours after sexual exposure but may be effective for up to 120 hours (off licence).
- It is thought to work primarily by inhibiting ovulation.
- There is no evidence that it is harmful in pregnancy and it can therefore be used if there have been other episodes of unprotected sexual intercourse earlier on in the menstrual cycle.
- It can be used more than once in a cycle.

Ulipristal acetate

- Ellaone® (Ulipristal acetate) was licensed in 2009 for emergency contraception.
- It is a progesterone receptor modulator and its primary mode of action is inhibition or delay of ovulation.
- Evidence suggests it can prevent ovulation after the luteinising hormone (LH) surge has started.
- It is licensed for use up to 120 hours after unprotected sexual intercourse.
- Its safety in pregnancy has not been established and therefore it cannot be used if there have been other episodes of unprotected sexual intercourse in the same cycle that were outside the 120 hour treatment window.
- It should not be used more than once in a cycle.

Testing for STIs (including HIV)

All victims should be offered testing for STIs, irrespective of whether penetrative assault has occurred. This is because patients may not recall or disclose fully, or may have had impaired consciousness. In the case of children, they may not fully understand or be able to express what has occurred. There is also some evidence that the rates of preexisting STIs are higher in victims.

When someone first presents, testing for the following should be offered: gonorrhoea, chlamydia, trichomonas, syphilis, HIV and hepatitis B (occasionally hepatitis C). Testing should be repeated at 2 weeks post-assault for gonorrhoea, chlamydia and trichomonas; at 6 weeks for HIV and syphilis; and at 3 months for HIV and Hepatitis B.

If a client declines swabs or declines them from certain orifices, their wishes should be respected. Self taken swabs should be offered in these circumstances and to those who would rather not be examined. Table 19.1 shows recommended screening tests.

Chain of evidence for STI samples

If specimen evidence is used in a court of law, its movements from source to laboratory to court must be clearly documented as an unbroken chain of evidence. In the laboratory, if the sample is split and aliquots are sent to different places, a new laboratory chain of evidence form must be completed for each aliquot. Once the specimen has been tested and analysed, the place and condition of storage must be documented. In a microbiology laboratory, other aspects of the management of the sample are also important, such as the need to freeze and the type of organism, if isolated. This must be overseen by a senior member of staff who can attend court if necessary. Generally, chain of evidence documentation is only used for people for whom the finding of an STI could be relevant in court (see Chapters 21–23 and the section on legal aspects later in this chapter).

Post-exposure prophylaxis

Prophylaxis against bacterial STIs can be offered following sexual assault. The advantages are reassurance, prevention of complications and confirmed treatment if the client does not attend follow-up. The disadvantages are anxiety and unnecessary treatment. If antibiotics are given without testing and the client had an STI prior to the sexual assault, partner notification cannot occur. If prophylaxis is given, it should cover gonorrhoea, chlamydia and *Trichomonas vaginalis*. The current recommended regime is a single dose of ceftriaxone 500 mg IM, azithromycin 1 g oral and metronidazole 2 g oral (see Cybulska *et al.*, 2012). Avoid giving oral antibiotics at the same time as oral emergency contraception to avoid the emergency contraception being vomited. Those given prophylaxis should be offered follow-up STI screening after treatment to exclude treatment failure or reinfection.

Table 19.1 Recommended screening tests and sites (only sites of penetration or attempted penetration need to be sampled).

	Chlamydia and gonorrhea – nucleic acid amplification test (NAAT)	*Neisseria gonorrhoeae* culture	Microscopy for Gram-negative intracellular diplococci	Vaginal wet slides for yeasts, bacterial vaginosis and *Trichomonas vaginalis* (plus culture for TV or DNA amplification, if available)
Asymptomatic women	Endocervix or self-taken vulvovaginal Rectum Pharynx			
Symptomatic women	Endocervix or self-taken vulvovaginal Rectum Pharynx	Endocervix or self-taken vulvovaginal Urethra Rectum Pharynx	Endocervix Urethra Rectum	Vulvovaginal
Asymptomatic men	Urine or urethra Rectum Pharynx	Urethra Rectum Pharynx	Urethra Rectum	
Symptomatic men	Urine or urethra Rectum Pharynx	Urethra Rectum Pharynx	Urethra Rectum	

HIV post-exposure prophylaxis following sexual exposure

Concerns about HIV following sexual assault are common. Actual acquisition is rare in the UK but much more common in some other countries, such as parts of sub-Saharan Africa, which have a high prevalence of both HIV and sexual assault. The risk for males who are raped is often especially high. Risks can relate to both the assault and the assailant(s) (see Box 19.3).

Box 19.3 HIV acquisition

High-risk assaults

- Forced anal intercourse.
- Defloration (virgin).
- Trauma.
- Where there is exposure to other STIs.
- Multiple assailants.

High-risk assailants

- Those known to have HIV (especially if untreated).
- Men who have sex with men.
- Those from high-prevalence areas, e.g. sub-Saharan Africa, East Asia, India, the Caribbean, parts of North and South America.

If the sexual assault occurred within the previous 72 hours, HIV post-exposure prophylaxis following sexual exposure (PEPSE) should be considered. PEPSE consists of a combination of antiretroviral drugs taken daily and continued for 28 days with support and monitoring.

There is a lack of conclusive data about efficacy. Some limited studies suggest that PEPSE can be effective but may cause side effects such as nausea and diarrhoea. The combination of side effects, psychological trauma following rape and an understandable reluctance to take medication that reminds them of the assault means that many people discontinue. The individual's risk of acquiring HIV can be estimated (see Box 19.4) and if it is relatively low, the harms of PEPSE may outweigh the potential benefits (see Table 19.2). Anal rape is divided into receptive (the individual's rectum being penetrated) and insertive (the individual penetrating someone else's rectum) as the risks of acquiring HIV are greater for receptive anal rape.

Box 19.4 Individual risk of HIV following sexual assault

If a woman was raped by an injecting drug user, the risk of acquiring HIV is estimated by multiplying *the assailant's risk of HIV* (~1 in 25) by *the risk of exposure* (1 in 600–2000 from an episode of vaginal intercourse, or higher if anal intercourse or trauma were factors). In this case, the risk would be 1 in 15 000–50 000.

The actual antiretrovirals used for PEPSE, and other aspects of guidance, vary by country. British HIV Association guidelines are used in the UK. SARCs and emergency departments should be able to make an initial assessment and provide 3–5 days of medication. Sexual health and genitourinary medicine clinics are usually responsible for the ongoing prescribing and monitoring of PEPSE.

Hepatitis B

It is rare to acquire hepatitis B following sexual assault in the UK. Hepatitis B vaccination is very safe, and if it is given within 6 weeks of the assault it may act as post-exposure prophylaxis (see Box 19.5).

Box 19.5 Risk factors for hepatitis B and indications for hepatitis B vaccine (data from Cybulska *et al.*, 2012)

- Assailant known to be a hepatitis B carrier.
- Assailant has risk factors (IV drug user, man who has sex with men, high-prevalence area).
- Anal rape.
- Trauma and bleeding.
- Multiple assailants.
- Client wishes to be vaccinated.
- Client not known to be immune to hepatitis following vaccination.

Psychosocial support

The psychological needs of those presenting should be assessed at the first and all subsequent visits, especially if they have a history of mental health problems, previous self-harm or a history of drug or alcohol abuse. Anxiety and depression are common following sexual assault. Some individuals go on to develop post-traumatic stress disorder (PTSD) (see Chapter 4). Self-harm

Table 19.2 Whether to use PEPSE following sexual assault.

	Assailant HIV positive	Assailant high risk	Assailant low risk
Receptive anal rape[*,†]	Recommended	Recommended	Consider
Vaginal rape	Recommended	Consider	Not recommended unless there is trauma or bleeding
Oral rape with ejaculation	Consider	Consider	Not recommended
Oral rape without ejaculation	Not recommended	Not recommended	Not recommended

[*]Unless there is trauma or bleeding
[†]for insertive anal rape see PEPSE guidelines

risk identification should be carried out, for example by asking, 'Have you ever hurt yourself?' and 'Do you feel you might hurt yourself?' Those at immediate risk of self-harm should be referred to emergency medical or acute mental health services urgently. Those at non-immediate risk should be referred to a health advisor, counsellor, psychologist or their GP. Many SARCs can also offer support. Even those who appear to have no psychological concerns should be given written information about appropriate organisations, such as rape crisis centres and the Samaritans, and should be offered follow-up in case of delayed presentation.

Early communication with the client's GP is very useful, if the client agrees to this. GPs may be able to offer ongoing support and referral to other services. They may also look after other family members who have been directly or indirectly affected.

Safety and child protection

Consideration should be given to clients' safety at home prior to their leaving the service, especially if the sexual assault was by someone known to them. It may be appropriate to help with finding a place of safety, rehousing or changing their mobile phone number. Child protection issues must be considered for any child or young person who has experienced or witnessed sexual assault or abuse or if there are concerns about a client's ability to look after their children (see Chapter 5).

Legal aspects of STIs and indication of sexual abuse or assault

The presence of an STI can be used as evidence in medicolegal cases. This is most likely if it is diagnosed in a child, a young person who has never been sexually active or someone who has not been sexually active for 5 or more years, or in a previously non-experienced site (e.g. in rectal swabs of someone who has not previously engaged in anal sex). In some cases it can link an assailant to a victim (e.g. through typing of gonorrhoea).

However, as an STI may have been present in the victim prior to assault, the usefulness in prosecution is limited. In some past cases the finding has been used against the victim.

The presence of an STI can be especially useful in prepubertal children. Interpretation of results requires expertise, as the type of test, risk of false positives and exclusion of vertical transmission or other nonsexual routes all need to be considered. However, any STI in a prepubertal child, including genital warts and bloodborne viruses, should be considered a possible indicator of child sexual abuse and expert opinion should be sought (Box 19.6).

Box 19.6 **STIs as a marker of sexual abuse in prepubertal children**

- Sexual abuse is the most likely mode of transmission for gonorrhoea, chlamydia and *Trichomonas vaginalis*. In such cases, urgent referral to child protection services is required.
- A significant proportion of children with anogenital warts have been sexually abused.

- For HIV infection and syphilis, child sexual abuse is likely if mother–child transmission (including breast feeding) and blood contamination have been excluded.
- For all STIs, a positive diagnosis in the mother does not exclude child sexual abuse.
- If the presence of an STI is to be used as evidence, the best possible test available must be used for diagnosis.
- Positive results on nucleic acid amplification tests (NAATs) should be confirmed using a different assay.

Further reading

Benn, P., Fisher, M., Kulasegaram, R. & BASHH (2011) PEPSE Guidelines Writing Group Clinical Effectiveness Group UK guideline for the use of post-exposure prophylaxis for HIV following sexual exposure. *International Journal of STD & AIDS*, **2011**, 695–708.

Cybulska, B., Forster, G., Welch, J., Lacey, H., Rogstad, K. & Lazaro, N. (2012) UK National Guidelines on Management of adult and adolescent complainants of sexual assault, http://www.bashh.org/documents/4450.pdf (last accessed 12 February 2014).

Cowling, P. (2008) *Guidelines for Handling Medicolegal Specimens and Preserving the Chain of Evidence.* Royal College of Pathologists, London.

Faculty of Sexual and Reproductive Healthcare (2012) *Faculty of Sexual and Reproductive Healthcare Guidance: Emergency Contraception. Clinical Effectiveness Unit*, http://www.fsrh.org/pdfs/CEUguidanceEmergency Contraception11.pdf (last accessed 12 February 2014).

Rogstad, K. (2011) *ABC of Sexually Transmitted Infections*, 6th Edition. John Wiley & Sons, Ltd, Chichester.

Royal College of Paediatrics and Child Health (2008) *The Physical Signs of Child Sexual Abuse: An Evidence-Based Review and Guidance for Best Practice*, http://www.rcpch.ac.uk/csa (last accessed 12 February 2014).

Useful contacts

Rape Crisis Centres, freephone 0808 802 99 99, www.rapecrisis.org.uk (last accessed 12 February 2014).

The NHS Choices Web site provides a postcode search for sexual violence services and SARCs, http://www.nhs.uk/Service-Search/Rape-and-sexual-assault-referral-centres/LocationSearch/364 (last accessed 12 February 2014).

The Samaritans (24 hour/day), 08457 90 90 90, www.samaritans.org (last accessed 12 February 2014).

Learning resources

Module on sexual abuse and assault, http://www.e-lfh.org.uk/projects/sexual-health-and-hiv/ (last accessed 12 February 2014).

Web site

Criminal Injuries Compensation Authority, http://www.justice.gov.uk/about/criminal-injuries-compensation-authority (last accessed 12 February 2014).

CHAPTER 20

Documenting in the Notes

Ali Mears

Genitourinary Medicine and HIV, Imperial College Healthcare NHS Trust, UK

OVERVIEW

- Documentation is an essential element of best clinical practice
- It should provide another person (or yourself at a future time) a snapshot understanding of what happened at the consultation, in terms of history, who was present, who said what, any physical findings (negative and positive), the management plan (including any concerns) and how any concerns were addressed
- The same factors apply to the alleged victim of sexual assault but there also are some specific additional ones to consider
- When a patient alleges assault, the best notes possible will help the doctor provide a statement or give evidence in court

Documentation of the history

All health care professionals are aware that clear and accurate contemporaneous documentation is an essential part of good patient care. Consultations with patients who have experienced physical or sexual assault are no exception. Indeed, it is more likely in such cases that a report or statement will be requested in the future. This is certainly the right time to demonstrate exemplary documentation skills.

You may be asked to provide a report for a criminal injuries compensation claim or a police statement, or you could find yourself in court as a professional witness. In addition, your notes may be requested for disclosure by the police, the Crown Prosecution Service or defence lawyers in civil or criminal cases.

In addition to the general principles of good documentation that you learn in basic training there are some extra skills and points you need to be aware of when documenting your consultation with an alleged victim of assault (see Box 20.1).

It is also important that you make a contemporaneous record of any telephone calls you receive or make regarding your patient and document clearly any advice you give or receive.

The history of the alleged assault is only part of the history taking. It is important to document all aspects just as rigorously, including the standard parts (past medical history, drug history etc.) and

anything more specific such as a mental health risk assessment that you carry out in the management of the patient.

Box 20.1 **History documentation – dos and don'ts**

Do

- Write contemporaneously – write notes at the time or immediately afterwards.
- Write legibly.
- Be objective and stick to the facts – avoid injudicious language.
- Explain the concept of confidentiality at the beginning of the consultation and that everything the patient tells you may be disclosable in court.
- Remember your role and only ask what you need to know about the assault to enable good management (concentrating on what was done, when, where and by whom).
- Record information from third parties as such: '*A.N. Other, staff nurse on X ward, told me that ...*'
- Record relevant information from the patient verbatim: '*He punched me twice in the face and my lip split.*'
- Sign all entries (sign and add your name afterwards in block capitals or with a name stamp).
- Date all entries (date and time).
- Document who else was present at the time of the consultation (or for a certain part of the consultation), e.g. mother, nurse, interpreter etc.
- Document a clear management plan.

Don't

- Leave documentation until the end of your shift.
- Think you are a police officer and start taking a detailed history that goes on for pages and pages (this might do the patient a real disservice if it contradicts a report given to the police).
- Ask leading questions.
- Be selective about what you write down – don't leave out a detail because you think it might 'sound bad' in court (remember you are not an investigator but simply a health care worker).
- Write illegibly or use nonapproved abbreviations (you will wish you could read what you wrote at 2 a.m. 2 years later when you are asked for a statement or find yourself being cross-examined by a barrister).

ABC of Domestic and Sexual Violence, First Edition.
Edited by Susan Bewley and Jan Welch.
© 2014 John Wiley & Sons, Ltd. Published 2014 by John Wiley & Sons, Ltd.

As outlined in the recent GMC guidance *Protecting Children and Young People: The Responsibilities of all Doctors* (General Medical Council, 2012), you must also record your concerns (including minor ones) and the details of any action you take. You must document clearly what information you have shared (if any, as well as why and with whom) and any decisions you have made relating to your concerns. For example, you may discover that a child has witnessed the assault of his or her mother or ongoing domestic violence, which will raise serious safeguarding concerns that you will need to deal with.

If a patient is referred to a sexual assault referral centre (SARC) for a forensic medical examination, the sexual offences examiner will undertake a very detailed history and examination on a pro forma that can span 30 or so pages. This type of examination (history, examination and DNA samples) does not occur elsewhere in medicine. This specific pro forma is not appropriate for other medical settings as the forensic role is very different. However, depending on which area of medicine you work in (e.g. A&E or genitourinary medicine), there may well be a specific brief pro forma that your department uses when seeing alleged victims of assault. Make sure you ask about this so that you use the correct paperwork.

More specific paperwork may be used by your department, such as a checklist for the management of victims of domestic violence or a more formal risk assessment such as an identification checklist. Make sure you are aware of, and follow, your department's guidelines.

Documenting physical findings

Chapters 12, 18 and 19 cover whether and when to examine an alleged victim of assault. When you do examine a patient in this situation, the documentation of physical findings needs to be as meticulous as that of the history.

As in any area of medicine, there is an accepted 'language'. For example, when describing an infected leg ulcer in a diabetic patient on hospital admission before starting antibiotics, your description must enable another member of the team who was not there at the time to understand what the ulcer looked like initially. Documentation of any physical injuries in an alleged victim of assault is no different. If you are asked to write a statement or are called to court to give evidence, you want to be confident that you can read and understand what you saw at 11.30 p.m. on a Saturday night 1 year previously and that you are using terms that all parties will understand (including the legal team and other professional or expert witnesses).

Thus, it is extremely important that you understand the 'language' when assessing someone for physical injuries: both what actual words and descriptions to use and, practically, how you should document these findings in a recognised way. The key elements of best practice are outlined in Box 20.2.

Box 20.2 Best practice when documenting physical findings

- Always use accepted descriptions (e.g. 'abrasion').
- Always use standard anatomical nomenclature (e.g. 'left iliac fossa' or 'posterior fourchette').
- Use anatomical body sketches or diagrams to record injuries.
- Measure the injury, mark it on the diagram and describe it clearly (e.g. 'round yellow bruise 2.8 × 2.8 cm, 5 cm above the olecranon, on the posterior aspect of the right arm'.)
- Take your time and document all findings as above.
- Some of your findings might be related to the assault and others might not. It is not for you to decide. Simply document what you see.
- Be aware that very often there are no physical injuries following sexual assault.
- Remember to also document the absence of injuries.

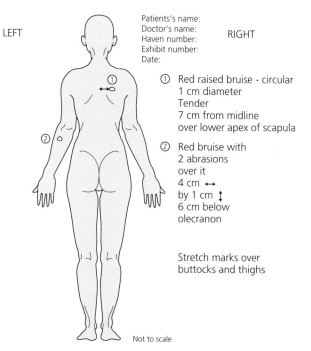

Patients's name:
Doctor's name:
Haven number:
Exhibit number:
Date:

LEFT

① Circular bruise - yellow
2.5 cm diameter
3 cm below
Acromioclavicular joint
Non tender

② Mole

③ Fresh red
non scabbed
abrasion
6 cm long
0.1 cm wide
12 cm above the
upper edge of right
patella

④ Tattoo

RIGHT

Not to scale

Patients's name:
Doctor's name:
Haven number:
Exhibit number:
Date:

LEFT   RIGHT

① Red raised bruise - circular
1 cm diameter
Tender
7 cm from midline
over lower apex of scapula

② Red bruise with
2 abrasions
over it
4 cm ↔
by 1 cm ↕
6 cm below
olecranon

Stretch marks over
buttocks and thighs

Not to scale

Figure 20.1 Forensic body diagram for use when documenting physical findings (with thanks to The Havens).

Box 20.3 explains the common nomenclature that you should use when describing an injury (see also Chapter 18). Be aware that very often there will be no physical injuries as a result of sexual assault. Remember when you examine a patient that it is also extremely important to document the *absence* of injuries.

Box 20.3 **Common accepted terms used to document injuries**

The following classification is used by forensic examiners. These are clear, simple terms that are recommended to everyone who documents injuries:

1 **Bruises:** Sometimes called 'contusions'.
2 **Abrasions:** Scratches, grazes, superficial injuries.
3 **Lacerations:** Cuts and tears caused by kicking or by weapons such as sticks or bottles.
4 **Incisions:** Clean-cut wounds made by a bladed weapon such as a knife.
5 **Stab wounds:** Penetrating wounds.
6 **Burns:** Wounds caused by extremes of temperature, electrical or chemicals.

Specialist forensic examiners use printed body diagrams when documenting their head-to-toe examination findings (see Figure 20.1). You do not need to worry if you do not have these (but please use them if you work in a department where they are available, such as A&E): you can simply draw the relevant area of the body in the notes and document your findings using the guidelines set out in the boxes found in this chapter.

Depending on your area of work, you may only infrequently see alleged victims of assault. Make sure you are familiar with what is expected from you in your role and document all findings carefully in the notes, in line with the advice in this chapter.

Further reading

British Association for Sexual Health and HIV (BASHH) (2011) *UK National Guidelines on the Management of Adult and Adolescent Complainants of Sexual Assault 2011*, http://www.bashh.org/documents/4450.pdf (last accessed 12 February 2014).

Coordinated Action Against Domestic Abuse (2012) CAADA-DASH Risk Identification Checklist (RIC) for MARAC Agencies, http://www.caada.org.uk/marac/RIC_without_guidance.pdf (last accessed 12 February 2014).

Faculty of Forensic and Legal Medicine (n.d.) Pro forma: examination of adult complainant of domestic violence, http://fflm.ac.uk/upload/documents/1289821108.pdf (last accessed 12 February 2014).

General Medical Council (2012) *Protecting Children and Young People: The Responsibilities of all Doctors*, http://www.gmc-uk.org/publications/13683.asp?dm_i=OUY,VFWP,3F73ZN,2LFC9,1 (last accessed 12 February 2014).

General Medical Council (2013) Good medical practice, http://www.gmc-uk.org/guidance/good_medical_practice.asp (last accessed 12 February 2014).

CHAPTER 21

Law and Prosecuting Practice in Relation to Serious Sexual Assaults and Domestic Violence

Wendy Cottee

Crown Prosecution Service, UK

OVERVIEW

- This chapter covers the prosecution process in England and Wales
- Sexual assault and the elements of specific sexual offences are defined
- Domestic violence covers a range of criminal behaviours and crimes
- Prosecutors benefit from clear and full notes
- Because of confidentiality, information sharing with third parties should be done with consent or after taking advice

The prosecution process in England and Wales

This chapter covers the legal process in England and Wales. The corresponding legislation elsewhere in the UK is set out in The Sexual Offences (Scotland) Act 2009 and the Sexual Offences (Northern Ireland) Order 2008. Other jurisdictions may have different legal processes and laws, with which you should familiarise yourself if necessary.

Criminal offences are investigated by the police. Evidence gathered by the police in relation to serious sexual assault cases and cases involving domestic violence is then passed to a lawyer from the Crown Prosecution Service (the organisation responsible for bringing criminal cases on behalf of the state). That lawyer will consider the evidence and advise the police as to any further evidence that needs to be obtained.

If there is sufficient evidence to give a realistic prospect of a successful prosecution and if a prosecution is in the public interest (it nearly always is in these cases) then the lawyer will decide what charges should be brought.

The defendant (the person charged) will then be charged and criminal court proceedings will commence. Figure 21.1 shows the progress of a case through court.

The lawyer from the Crown Prosecution Service will then prepare the case for court. Usually a separate lawyer will be responsible for

Arrest/Court Process

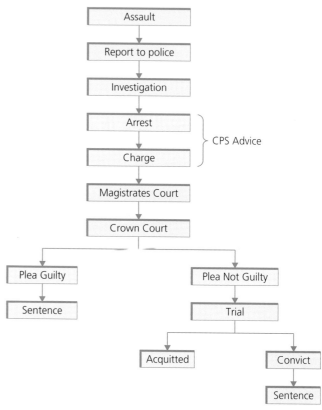

Figure 21.1 The arrest and court process (with thanks to The Havens).

the presentation of the court case. Lawyers and police work together on the preparation and presentation of the case.

A defendant will also be represented by a lawyer in court. The English court system is an adversarial one, which means that each party presents evidence in court and it is then challenged by the opposing party. Box 21.1 shows the likely types of evidence to be brought to court.

ABC of Domestic and Sexual Violence, First Edition.
Edited by Susan Bewley and Jan Welch.
© 2014 John Wiley & Sons, Ltd. Published 2014 by John Wiley & Sons, Ltd.

What is a sexual assault?

A sexual assault is any act which by its nature or purpose would appear to be sexual and to which, in the case of adults, there is no freely given consent.

Children under the age of 16 years are deemed in law not to be able to consent to sexual activity. Therefore, any sexual act with a person under 16 is a sexual offence. Where the parties are around the same age and the sex is in effect consensual it is unlikely any prosecution would be brought.

The majority of sexual offences are governed by the Sexual Offences Act 2003, which came into force on 1 May 2004. Any offence committed since that date will be governed by this Act.

The Act deals with a vast range of sexual offences and creates separate offences against adults and children. It offers protection to children not only from sexual acts but also from preparatory offences such as sexual grooming. There are specific offences that offer protection to vulnerable adults against sexual assaults from those in a position of trust, such as care workers (see Chapter 14). There are also protections for adults with a mental or physical disability as a result of which they cannot freely consent to any sexual act. The three most common adult offences are explained in Box 21.2.

Box 21.2 **Most common adult offences under the Sexual Offences Act 2003**

Rape (Section 1)

The elements of rape are that:

- A (the perpetrator/defendant) intentionally penetrates the vagina, anus or mouth of another person B with his penis;
- B does not consent to the penetration; and
- A does not reasonably believe that B consents.

Note the perpetrator has to be male, as penetration by a penis is the prerequisite of the offence.

The complainant B can be male or female, as penetration of the mouth and anus are both rape.

Rape can take place even if the parties are married if B does not freely consent to the sexual activity.

The fact that A was so drunk he did not know what he was doing is no defence to any sexual offence.

Note that if B was under the influence of drink or drugs at the time of any sexual act it may be the case that he or she was then unable to freely consent to the act. It is therefore important when dealing with patients who may have been sexually assaulted to ascertain whether this is the case and obtain blood or urine samples, which may assist in any prosecution.

Rape carries a maximum penalty of life imprisonment and can only be tried in a crown court.

Assault by penetration (Section 2)

A person (A) commits this offence if:

- He/she intentionally penetrates the vagina or anus of another person B with a part of his/her body or anything else;
- That act of penetration is sexual;
- B does not consent to the penetration; and
- A does not reasonably believe that B consents.

The penetration has to be of the vagina or anus, but unlike rape this is not a gender-specific offence – a male or a female can commit it against a male (penetration of anus) or a female (penetration of anus or vagina).

The part of A's body might be, for example, a finger or toe or the tongue.

'Anything else' is literally that (e.g. a bottle).

This offence is often charged where the victim B does not know whether the penetration was by a penis or something else.

Like rape, assault by penetration is punishable with a maximum of life imprisonment and can only be tried in a crown court.

Sexual assault (Section 3)

A person (A) commits this offence if:

- He/she intentionally touches another person B;
- The touching is sexual;
- B does not consent to the touching; and
- A does not reasonably believe that B consents.

There is an overlap between this offence and S2 above, as it can include penetration.

Touching can be with a part of A's body or with anything else. It does not need to be skin-on-skin touching but can be through/over clothing.

The touching must be of a sexual nature, which is determined by the circumstances of the touching and the purpose of A in doing it. For example, an intimate medical examination will by its circumstances appear sexual but the purpose of the examination is a proper one and would not therefore be sexual touching (so long as there is consent).

This is not a gender-specific offence: a person of either sex can commit it.

Domestic violence

There is no specific statutory offence of domestic violence but the government definition is 'any incident of threatening behaviour, violence or abuse (psychological, physical, sexual, financial or emotional) between adults who are or have been intimate partners of family members, regardless of gender or sexuality' (Home Office, 2013).

It can refer to physical, sexual, or emotional abuse, including physical assaults, sexual assaults and harassment, and also covers female genital mutilation, forced marriage and so-called 'honour crimes'.

If a man punches a woman for no reason that is an assault. If that woman is his wife or partner then it is still an assault but it will be termed 'domestic violence'. This is an aggravating feature that will serve to increase the normal sentence for this type of offence.

What to do if your patient may be the victim of a sexual assault or domestic violence

- Make clear and full notes of the examination and any injuries found – include full body diagrams of any injuries (see Chapters 18 and 20).
- Fully note anything said by the victim about how the injuries were caused and what happened.
- If there is evidence of the influence of drink or drugs, try and obtain urine/blood samples.
- Encourage reporting to the police.
- These offences are often about control, so ensure that the victim is seen independently from anyone who may be either the perpetrator of the offence or a supporter of the same, who will not allow the victim to speak freely (e.g. a victim of domestic violence escorted to hospital by a partner who has assaulted her).
- Consider referral to support organisations.

The prosecution approach to cases of sexual assault and domestic violence

These types of case are taken very seriously by police and prosecutors alike.

Only specially trained lawyers and advocates can deal with rape and serious sexual offences. Likewise, all prosecutors receive detailed training in dealing with cases of domestic violence.

Victims of sexual offences have a right to lifetime anonymity in respect of the allegation. Various so-called 'special measures' are available to assist victims through the process of giving evidence in court so as to ensure that they are protected and supported and thus to enable them to give the best possible evidence. These measures include giving evidence by way of video-recorded interview and being able to answer questions through a video link, in order to prevent the trauma of going into the courtroom. Alternatively, the victim can choose to be screened from the defendant when in court so that during the process of giving evidence he/she does not have to see the defendant.

Questioning of victims about past sexual history is generally not permitted. While there are some exceptions to this, the questioning is strictly supervised by the trial judge. The defendant can only ask questions of a victim of sexual assault or domestic violence through his/her lawyer and not in person.

Confidentiality and information sharing

In general, doctors should protect patients' confidentiality and not give any details to any third parties without consent. What is the legal status of the medical notes of a victim of a sexual or domestic assault?

The general rule is that there is no such thing as confidentiality in relation to the medical notes of a victim of sexual/domestic assault when the matter reaches the criminal courts (i.e. at the subpoena stage). Those victims seen at a specialist sexual assault examination centre will sign a pro forma to indicate they understand this. Police will also explain this to any victim of such assaults.

If a defendant charged with a sexual offence indicates to the court that he/she will be pleading not guilty, a process called 'disclosure' is triggered: the prosecution is obliged to disclose any information of which it is aware that either undermines the prosecution case or assists the defendant's case. Medical notes may come within this category. These cannot be disclosed without the consent of the victim, but if this is withheld it can jeopardise the prosecution case.

There are, however, many incidents where past medical history will simply not be relevant to the case and need not be disclosed to the defence.

Any disputes in relation to what can be disclosed are determined by the trial judge before the trial commences.

The most important thing to remember is that, as stated before, all details of examination findings and remarks made by the patient should be fully noted and disclosed to the police with the patient's consent when requested. If you have any doubts about breaches of confidentiality or your position, discuss these with a senior doctor or your medical defence organisation.

Further reading

Crown Prosecution Service (2013) *Code for Crown Prosecutors*, http://www.cps.gov.uk/publications/code_for_crown_prosecutors/ (last accessed 12 February 2014).

Crown Prosecution Service (no date) *CPS Policy for Prosecuting Cases of Domestic Violence*, http://www.cps.gov.uk/publications/prosecution/domestic/domv.html (last accessed 12 February 2014).

Home Office (2013) Circular: new government domestic violence and abuse definition, https://www.gov.uk/government/publications/new-government-domestic-violence-and-abuse-definition (last accessed 12 February 2014).

CHAPTER 22

Writing a Statement as a Professional Witness

Bernadette Butler

The Haven Camberwell Sexual Assault Referral Centre, King's College Hospital NHS Foundation Trust, UK

OVERVIEW

- Clinicians may be required to provide a statement in relation to an investigation
- This may be used in court proceedings
- It is important to establish for what investigation or court it is required
- The clinician has an overriding duty to tell the truth and an obligation to assist the court
- The statement relates to their professional work
- It must be written so that it is objective, clear, unambiguous and understandable by readers (most of whom will have no clinical background)

Introduction

A clinician may attend court in a number of roles (see Box 22.1).

Box 22.1 Clinician attendance at court

- **Witness of fact:** Giving information about something seen or heard, or in which the individual was involved.
- **Professional witness:** Giving information in the context of their professional role, e.g. doctor, nurse, paramedic. Doctors might include some explanation or interpretation.
- **Expert witness:** Where the statement will be based on other information provided, partially or completely outwith the direct involvement of the clinician, and will include interpretation, comment and opinion.
- **Defendant:** In a civil or criminal case.

This chapter deals only with professional witness statements. These may be needed for:

- The criminal courts, e.g. magistrate's court, crown court.
- The coroner's court.

Similarly, reports, rather than statements, may be needed for other proceedings, such as the family court; these are not covered here.

ABC of Domestic and Sexual Violence, First Edition.
Edited by Susan Bewley and Jan Welch.
© 2014 John Wiley & Sons, Ltd. Published 2014 by John Wiley & Sons, Ltd.

A statement is essentially a formal account of the facts relating to an incident or occurrence (see Box 22.2). It is usually a document written by the clinician. Sometimes it is given orally and written down by a police officer; the witness is then asked to read it, make any amendments, initial them and sign it. If an oral statement is given, it must be read and edited carefully before signature, as the duties and obligations still apply.

Box 22.2 What do I do when I am asked to write a statement?

- Don't panic.
- Check the request is in writing.
- Confirm (if not already clarified):
  - *About whom* it is to be written and *what event(s)* it should cover, e.g. a patient you saw in the A&E on a particular day.
  - *By whom* it is needed, e.g. police.
  - The *time frame* within which it is required, e.g. for a hearing next month.
- Acknowledge the request and explain any likely delay, e.g. if you are going on annual leave.
- Don't be rushed – a quality document requires time to prepare and write.

Criminal justice procedures and laws differ between and within countries:

- In the UK, there are differences between procedures in England & Wales and those in Scotland and Northern Ireland.
- In other countries, there may be differences between state and federal legislation.
- It is important to know where you can get advice if you are uncertain (e.g. professional and medical indemnity organisations).

Purpose

The statement should assist an investigation and the court by proving an account of your involvement; that is, what was:

- Seen.
- Said and heard.
- Done.

Or a combination of all of these.

Witness Statement
(CJ Act 1967, s9 MC Act 1980, ss. 5A (3) (a) and 5B; MC Rules 1981,r. 70)
Statement of: Dr Iama Medic MB BS
Age (if under 18): Over 18 (if over 18 insert 'over 18')
Occupation: Registered Medical Practitioner (Hospital Doctor)
This statement (consisting of 1 page signed by me) is true to the best of my knowledge and belief and I make it knowing that, if it is tendered in evidence, I shall be liable to prosecution if I have wilfully stated anything which I know to be false or do not believe to be true.

Date: 1 April 2014   Signature: *Iama Medic*

---

1 Introduction

This is a professional witness statement requested by PC Cop of Anyshire Police about my examination of Snow White (SW) on 31 December 2013 and is based on my contemporaneous notes.

2 Author

My name is Dr Iama Medic. I graduated as Bachelor of Medicine (MB) and Bachelor of Surgery (BS) from the University of Anycity in 2009. I am a fully registered doctor with the General Medical Council (GMC), Registration Number: XXXXXXX. I am a First-Year Specialty Trainee (ST1) in General Practice and my current post is at Anyshire University Hospital in the Emergency Department (ED), which I started on 1 December 2013.

3 The statement

3.1 Background

On Friday 31 December 2013, at 21:00, I was on duty at Anyshire University Hospital when I attended to Snow White (SW), aged 21 years (DOB: 1/1/1992) in the resuscitation area of the ED. SW was given a reference number: ED0123456.

3.2 The history, examination and findings.

3.2.1 SW had arrived by ambulance, with two others, who said their names were Grumpy and Happy and that they were SW's house mates.

3.2.2 SW appeared very short of breath (dyspnoeic), she was coughing and her breathing was noisy; initially she could not speak, but pointed to her mouth and throat. Her lips were blue (cyanosed) and she was distressed.

3.2.3 The ambulance crew, Jakob and William Grimm, told me they attended SW's house at 20:45 on 31/12/13, following a '999' call, and found her to be very short of breath. Grumpy and Happy said she had choked on an apple. The Grimms told me they had tried the usual treatments: back slaps and the Heimlich manoeuvre (an upwards thrust just beneath the front of the ribcage) to try and force the obstruction out. These failed, so they had:

- Given SW oxygen by mask.
- Put up a drip (obtained intravenous access) and given fluids.
- Attached a small device (pulse oximeter), which measured the oxygen in the blood: the level (saturation) was 84% (low).
- Transported her to hospital, using the ambulance's blue light and siren.

3.2.4 It is my normal practice to take a history and examine the patient, but in emergency situations the usual sequence may be altered.

3.2.5 I continued the oxygen (O_2) at 15 litres per minute and checked the oximetry reading, which was still 84%.

3.2.6 SW's blood pressure was 90/60 mm of mercury (normal) and her pulse was 140 beats per minute (very fast). Grumpy and Happy told me they had not seen what happened but believed SW had been forced to eat an apple by her stepmother and a piece had 'gone down the wrong way'; it seemed this had entered her trachea (windpipe), causing a partial obstruction.

3.2.7 I decided to try back slaps again. I explained this to SW, who nodded; I took this as consent. At 21:15, on the second slap, SW gave a huge cough and a piece of apple was propelled from her mouth. Her breathing settled to normal within a few minutes; she was not distressed and her O_2 saturation returned to 99% (normal).

3.2.8 I obtained a history from SW. She said that while eating an apple, a bit went down the wrong way and she could not cough it back up, and she became breathless. She said she was healthy and had never been in hospital. She took no medicines and had no allergies.

3.2.9 I completed my examination of SW. There were two blue bruises, each 1 cm in diameter, overlying the right and left angles of her jaw (mandible).

3.2.10 I noted two blue/purple bruises on the back (dorsum) of both wrists, each 1.2 cm in diameter. The bruises were overlying the wrist creases, centrally, 2 cm from the bony prominence at the wrist (ulnar styloid).

3.2.11 I asked SW what caused these bruises; she said they were from doing housework and had been there for several days. When I asked more questions, she said: 'I am sure they are from housework. I don't want to talk about them. Grumpy and Happy got it wrong; my stepmother wasn't there when I ate the apple.'

3.2.12 The examination was otherwise unremarkable (normal). There was no need for further tests.

3.2.13 At 22:45, I discharged SW, but advised her to return if there was any problem. I believe she left with Grumpy and Happy. I have not seen SW since.

4 Summary

4.1 SW presented after inhaling a piece of apple.

4.2 She had bruises on her face and wrists, which she said were from housework.

Date: 1 April 2014   Signature: *Iama Medic*

Figure 22.1 Sample witness statement (fictional).

If a clinician writes a statement using another's notes or records, this must be made clear.

Duties and obligations

You have an overriding duty to tell the truth and an obligation to assist the court.

You may have a declaration to make at the beginning or the end of the document. There may be a mandatory form of words for the jurisdiction in which you work.

It is important to note that if you do not fulfil your duties and obligations, your probity, and in turn your fitness to practice, may be called into question.

Do I need the patient's permission to write a statement?

It depends. You may have written confirmation of the patient's permission but you should clarify this. Discuss the statement with a senior colleague, the legal department or the information governance lead in your trust and/or your professional indemnity organisation. Check whether there is a local policy or protocol to which you should refer. Some criminal and statutory investigations may require you to comply with such a request whether or not you have the patient's permission to do so.

How do I start?

1 Ask your clinical supervisor or a senior colleague for advice; there may be a 'local' template to use.
2 Look at examples written by experienced colleagues.
3 Obtain the relevant notes or records.
4 Set aside the time – at least 2 hours.
5 Avoid interruptions (do not write a statement when on duty).
6 Read everything several times, before you start.
7 Plan the layout, if you do not have a template.

What do I do next?

1 Decide what information should be included (a template will help; see Figure 22.1 and Box 22.3).
2 Start writing – computers make editing easier.
3 Be objective and accurate.
4 Use a clear, suitably sized font.
5 Consider double line spacing.
6 Number the pages and paragraphs. This makes it easy for the reader – which might be you in court later.
7 Double check the grammar, punctuation and spelling.

Box 22.3 **What should be in the statement?**

1 The date it was written.
2 The subject of, or reason for, the statement and the circumstances.
3 Brief details about yourself (name and qualification, regulatory body number), your experience and the nature of your role at the time of your involvement with the patient/incident.
4 Details of the patient – name, date of birth and the circumstances of presentation.
5 Anyone else present or involved, e.g. a parent, an interpreter, members of staff.
6 Who told you what – it must be clear what you were told directly and what others reported (hearsay). Consider including verbatim comments, such as 'My husband punched me'.
7 What you did and found (and sometimes what you did not do and did not find).
8 The end of your involvement.
9 A summary or conclusion.
10 If appropriate, an interpretation of your findings – but don't step beyond your area or level of knowledge or experience.
11 Use appendices, e.g. for body maps, x-ray reports.
12 Ensure any medical terms are explained either within the statement or as a glossary.

'Medical speak', jargon and acronyms must be explained (or avoided). On the one hand, you must communicate to a 'lay audience' (police, lawyers, judge, jury), rather as you would a patient, but on the other, your statement may be read by other clinicians who expect the 'professional' aspect. In a long report, consider a glossary, as it is essential all medical and scientific terms are clarified, as those who may read your statement may have no science education beyond secondary school level.

When it is ready, what do I do?

1 Read, check for spelling and typographical errors, and check again. Ensure the spell-check program is set up for the correct region (e.g. UK or US English) and that the spelling of a word is appropriate to its (not it's) context.
2 It is important to have a high level of attention to detail, as this reflects upon your credibility – you may need to ask for help with spelling and punctuation.
3 Reading a statement aloud will help you find errors.
4 Ask a senior colleague to check over your statement, but remember that it is *your* statement, so write only what you would feel confident repeating in court. Check whether your organisation requires a statement to be reviewed before it is released.
5 Print (single sided).

6 Sign and date.

7 Check whether another individual's signature is required.

8 Provide your contact details and dates when you are unavailable to attend court ('dates to avoid'). Make sure these are kept up to date.

9 Ensure there is a secure means of delivery and confirmation of receipt.

Summary

Witness statements are clearly very important, but with appropriate care and planning, advice, support and practice, you should be able to provide a good-quality, fit-for-purpose document that can assist the court. You may wish to attend training to improve your skills.

Further reading

Franklin, P.J. (2009) The doctor in court. In: McLay, W.D.S. (ed.) *Clinical Forensic Medicine*. Cambridge University Press, Cambridge, pp. 44–47.

General Medical Council (2009) *Confidentiality*, http://www.gmc-uk.org /static/documents/content/Confidentiality_0910.pdf (last accessed 12 February 2014).

General Medical Council (2013) *Acting as a witness in legal proceedings* http://www.gmc-uk.org/Acting_as_a_witness.pdf_51448308.pdf (last accessed 12 February 2014).

Parker, H.L. (2004) Writing a police statement. *Australian Family Physician*, **33**(11), 927–930.

Sakr, M. & Boyle, A., for the Clinical Effectiveness Committee of the College of Emergency Medicine (2012) Providing a witness statement for the police, http://www.collemergencymed.ac.uk/Shop-Floor/Clinical%20 Guidelines/Clinical%20Guidelines/ (last accessed 12 February 2014).

For help with writing your statement

Fowler, F. (2003) *A Dictionary of Modern English Usage*. Oxford University Press, Oxford – First published in 1829, this is the definitive style guide to British English usage, pronunciation and writing.

Truss, L. (2003) *Eats, Shoots & Leaves: The Zero Tolerance Guide to Punctuation*. Profile Books, London – An amusing and educational guide to punctuation.

CHAPTER 23

Going to Court

Bernadette Butler

The Haven Camberwell Sexual Assault Referral Centre, King's College Hospital NHS Foundation Trust, UK

OVERVIEW

- Clinicians may be required to give evidence in court
- This can be daunting but you are not on trial
- Preparation beforehand is essential
- Speak clearly and answer questions that are within your knowledge
- Do not be afraid to say, 'I don't know'
- Media representations of court are not often accurate

As a clinician you may be called to give evidence (see Box 23.1) in a variety of courts. Most commonly this will be in:

- A magistrates' court.
- A higher court (e.g. a crown court).
- A coroner's court.

Box 23.1 **What should I do when I get a court warning or notification to attend?**

1 Don't panic.
2 Confirm receipt and ask that you be contacted if there any changes; keep the contact details of the witness care unit or police officer-in-the-case.
3 If you are unavailable, tell the witness care unit or the officer-in-the-case immediately.
4 Check you have the correct details, e.g. the name of patient/case, the address of the court and the date of the trial/hearing. Note that the warning may only contain details of the defendant (e.g. 'The Crown'/'State vs Mr Q'), not those of the person whom you examined.
5 Make sure you have the date in your personal diary and that of the department, in case a locum is required or clinics need to be altered.
6 Tell your clinical supervisor or a senior colleague.
7 Consider speaking to your professional indemnity organisation.

Usually you will already have provided a witness statement (see Chapter 22). It is said that 'if you write a good statement, you won't

be called to court'. This is unhelpful, as it implies that if you are called, your statement was of poor quality. It is also incorrect, as there are numerous reasons why you might be called.

Court procedures are generally 'adversarial' or 'inquisitorial'. What you say in court is unlikely to be affected by this distinction, since your overriding duty is to assist the court, not to support the 'side' by whom you are called.

When you provide your statement, include dates on which you are unavailable to attend and keep these up to date. You must be aware that you might be called to court. If you do not attend when required, this can result in significant and serious consequences for you: a reprimand, a fine or even custody, if you are found guilty of contempt of court.

Preparation

By failing to prepare, you are preparing to fail
Benjamin Franklin, 1706–1790

Read through your statement and contemporaneous notes several times. Make a copy to take with you. Consider highlighting areas that you will want to find easily, such as the patient's name, dates and times and so on. Think how to explain findings and conditions, as well as what you might be asked and how you will answer (but don't worry if your predictions aren't fulfilled).

Make the most of the witness care unit or liaison services. They are there for *all* witnesses: tell them if you have not been to court before or have any particular requirements (e.g. wheelchair access). Ask if you can visit the court ahead of time to see its layout; you may not be able to visit the court in which the trial or hearing is to take place, but taking a look around a different one will give you an idea of what to expect.

On the day the trial starts

Although trials are listed to last a few days, clinicians are rarely needed at 9.00 a.m. on the first day: check with the witness care unit or the police officer-in-the-case.

What to take with you

1 A copy of your statement and notes, in a file.
2 Your spectacles, if you need them.
3 Some form of identification, such as a hospital badge.

ABC of Domestic and Sexual Violence, First Edition.
Edited by Susan Bewley and Jan Welch.
© 2014 John Wiley & Sons, Ltd. Published 2014 by John Wiley & Sons, Ltd.

4 The witness care unit and officer-in-the-case's contact numbers.
5 Something to occupy you while you are waiting, such as a news-paper.

What else should you do?

1 Dress in comfortable, smart clothes and shoes – look 'professional'.
2 Avoid caffeine and try to keep calm.
3 Leave plenty of time to get to court.
4 Let the witness care unit or officer-in-the-case know when you arrive: they will show you where to wait, either outside the court or in a private witness sitting room.
5 Remember that you should not talk to other witnesses about the case or your evidence.
6 Check your appearance: tidy your hair, straighten your tie, check your buttons and zips, take a 'comfort break'.

Before you go into court

1 A member of the legal team may speak to you.
2 Speak to the usher, who may be able to show you the court's layout.
3 Ask how you should address the judge, magistrate or coroner and about any court etiquette or protocol.
4 Confirm whether you want to take the oath on a holy book (and which one) or if you want to affirm (nonreligious).
5 Switch off your mobile phone or pager or put it on 'silent' – and then double check that you have!

When you go in

An oft-used adage is, 'Stand up, speak up and shut up'. Essentially this means: look professional, appear confident and capable (but not arrogant), make sure your audience can hear you and do not answer questions that are not within your knowledge or field (see Figure 23.1 and Box 23.2).

> Box 23.2 **Keep to your area of knowledge and expertise**
>
> *It is better to keep your mouth closed and let people think you are a fool than to open it and remove all doubt.*
>
> Mark Twain, 1835–1910

You may feel uncomfortable in a situation in which you perceive yourself as having little control and being under scrutiny. Even if you don't feel it, try to appear confident – after all, you were the one who saw the patient and did the examination, and only you can explain it to others.

Usually you will be shown to the witness box. You may stand or sit (most people stand). You will probably be asked to make a declaration, oath or affirmation. The words are usually provided on a card, along with a holy book if appropriate. Take a deep breath and read the words out in a measured way, *directing your gaze and words to the jury and/or the judge*. This conveys that you are trustworthy and that what you say is reliable.

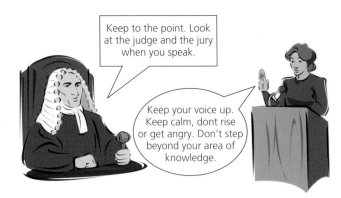

Figure 23.1 Top tips from experienced colleagues.

The questions

These almost always cover what you have written in your statement. They may be from more than one judicial officer. For example, you may be questioned first by the prosecution and then by the defence and/or the judge. In England and Wales, this is described as 'examination in chief' and 'cross-examination', respectively. If the prosecution then has further things to clarify, this is referred to as 'reexamination'.

In a coroner's court, there are 'properly interested parties', such as the family, who may have their own legal representative asking questions in addition to the coroner.

Lawyers know how uncomfortable court can be for a witness. They will often start with a 'setting the scene' approach, asking you your name, qualifications and experience before moving on to the pertinent matter: 'Let us now turn to the events of 31 December 2013, when I believe you examined Ms A at Anyshire Hospital.' It is usually OK to refer to your notes and statement. If this has not been confirmed, ask the judge.

- *Speak slowly and clearly* Notes will be taken, either by hand or on a computer. Another adage is, 'Watch the judge's pen' (or laptop).
- *Think before answering* Remember, you are there to help the court. Silence can be uncomfortable, but you must be accurate in your replies. If the answer is yes, say 'Yes' or 'That's correct'. If the answer is no, say 'No'. However, if the answer is not yes or no but needs qualification, you must provide it. If you do not understand the question, for example if there are two negatives or several questions at once, say so. Ask that the questions be repeated, or asked one at a time.
- *Do not be afraid to say, 'I don't know'* You can't know everything. Similarly, stay within your area of knowledge and expertise. If you know all there is to know, for example about pulse oximetry or bruising, then if asked, you should answer. On the other hand, if you don't know, stop when you reach the limit of your knowledge and say so. In an effort to be helpful, you may find yourself trying to answer questions that are outwith your knowledge or expertise.
- *Do not get angry or take it personally* Remember that the process is about scrutiny – 'testing' the evidence. Despite media portrayals of court, personal attacks and 'badgering' rarely happen. However, should you feel attacked and the judge does not intervene, you can ask for assistance: 'My Lord, I have answered this question to the best of my ability and I do not have anything more to add.'

Once you have finished giving evidence, you will be told if you may leave, and usually you will be thanked. You may be warned not to talk to anyone else about the case until the trial or hearing is concluded.

What do I do afterwards?

1 Relax, it's over.
2 Speak to the witness care unit about expenses – you or your organisation may be able to claim a fee for your time or towards the cost of a locum.
3 Try not to have too much of an immediate 'post mortem' on the events, but reflect on them later. You will often think of something you might have done differently, if not necessarily better.
4 Ask the witness care unit or officer-in-the-case to let you know the outcome (verdict and sentence). If it is not as you expected, do not assume responsibility – your role is just part of the picture.
5 You may want to consider some formal training – a witness or court skills course.
6 Peer review meetings where experiences are shared (but cases yet to go to trial are not discussed) can be of use in thinking about issues and preparing to give evidence.

Conclusion

During his or her professional working life, a clinician may have to give objective and impartial evidence in court or at a tribunal. With preparation, support and training, this can be achieved without anxiety. Some will so enjoy the process that their career development will include an active medicolegal role.

Further reading

Franklin, P.J. (2009). The doctor in court. In: McLay, W.D.S. (ed.) *Clinical Forensic Medicine*. Cambridge University Press, Cambridge, pp. 44–47.

Ministry of Justice (2008) The witness charter: standards of care for witnesses in the criminal justice system. http://www.justice.gov.uk /downloads/victims-and-witnesses/working-with-witnesses/witness -charter.pdf (last accessed 12 February 2014).

Robinson, S. (2004) Healthcare professionals in court – professional and expert witnesses. In: Payne-James, J., Wall, I. & Dean, P. (eds) *Medicolegal Essentials in Healthcare*. Cambridge University Press, Cambridge, pp. 233–240.

CHAPTER 24

Violation of Professional Boundaries

Fiona Subotsky

Royal College of Psychiatrists, UK

OVERVIEW

- Physical, sexual and emotional violence take place in health care settings
- Doctors can be perpetrators or victims, witnesses or unaware
- Patients are most vulnerable when least powerful
- Institutions and systems often resist complaints
- Doctors and other health care professionals need to be aware of their own susceptibility
- They must be prepared to take appropriate action when concerned by what they see or hear

---

Introduction

To become a doctor, one has to unlearn many cultural taboos. Doctor–patient encounters present situations of unusual intimacy, which might in other circumstances be connected with sexual attraction, and patients are both emotionally and physically vulnerable.

It has always been recognised that this can lead to risky situations. The Hippocratic oath included the following: 'Into as many houses as I enter, I will go for the benefit of the ill, while being far from all voluntary and destructive injustice, especially from sexual acts both upon women's bodies and upon men's, both of the free and of slaves.'

Rules and regulations

Rules about what constitutes inappropriate 'sexualised' behaviour have become clearer over recent years and include:

- *Contractual* Trust policies.
- *Professional* General Medical Council (GMC) Good Medical Practice standards.
- *Legal* Criminal law.

Each of these areas has its own investigative procedures and sanctions.

Are there risky (or at-risk) doctors?

The prevalence of sexual boundary violation among doctors is extremely difficult to establish, but mainly USA-based surveys and disciplinary findings suggest it is not uncommon. Doctors who break boundaries are more likely to be male and older, sometimes in powerful senior positions. The specialities most likely to be involved are general practice, psychiatry and obstetrics and gynaecology (see Boxes 24.1 and 24.2).

Box 24.1 Case study: Clifford Ayling, General Practitioner

Clifford Ayling worked in Kent as a GP and part-time clinical assistant in obstetrics and gynaecology, and also did family planning sessions. In 1998 he was arrested and charged with indecent assault of patients and was found guilty on 12 counts, for which he was imprisoned and struck off by the GMC in 1999. The incidents were generally of inappropriate touching or examination of women's breasts or genitals. There had been complaints for many years, which were not responded to effectively. The defence was that these were justified examinations, if old-fashionedly thorough.

The inquiry particularly recommended further advice on the use of chaperones and guidance on responding to 'sexualised behaviour' (Department of Health, 2004).

Box 24.2 Case study: William Kerr, Consultant Psychiatrist

Concerns were raised throughout his career … The allegations were of unscheduled domiciliary visits, or appointments being arranged for the end of clinics when there would be few nursing staff around. William Kerr would then allegedly expose himself and 'invite' patients to perform sexual acts (often of masturbation or oral sex) upon him, sometimes suggesting that this was part of their treatment. A number of patients also alleged that full sexual intercourse took place. A number of women described William Kerr's ability to make them comply with his wishes, leaving them confused and guilty about their own actions and afraid to complain … prior to 1983, of the 30 concerns alleged to have been raised about William Kerr all but one fell on deaf ears.

The Kerr/Haslam Inquiry, Department of Health (2005)

ABC of Domestic and Sexual Violence, First Edition.
Edited by Susan Bewley and Jan Welch.
© 2014 John Wiley & Sons, Ltd. Published 2014 by John Wiley & Sons, Ltd.

While the serial predator with psychopathic personality hits the headlines, 'single victim' cases are more common. A doctor may be convinced he is in love or that the emotional relationship will be therapeutic.

An awareness of general vulnerability is most useful.

Are there risky (or at-risk) patients?

Most obviously, vulnerable patients are the most powerless – such as children, the learning disabled and the mentally ill. However, it is easy to think in opposed stereotypes: the patient as innocent young female victim of a predatory and deceitful male doctor, or the foolish young doctor falling prey to a seductive woman who has demanded a late home visit. These situations certainly arise, but there are also more nuances, and many exceptions (see Box 24.3). Same-sex incidents can occur, and a patient may well have previous experience of sexual abuse, making her or him vulnerable.

Box 24.3 **Case study: whose slippery slope?**

A male doctor, Dr A, gave a female patient, Ms B, a lift to the station. It had been the last appointment of the day and it was pouring with rain. Two weeks later the patient makes another late appointment, and suggests a drink together on the way home.

- Should the doctor have offered a lift in the first place?
- What should he say now?
- What difference do age and gender make to this scenario?

Dr A puts Ms B off and mentions the incident in a passing, jokey way to a colleague, Dr C, a trainee with the practice. This is overheard by the receptionist, Ms D.

- How might Dr C and Ms D feel about this?
- Do they have any responsibilities?

A month later, Ms B makes another appointment with Dr A, who feels uncomfortable over whether there is a real medical need but tries to remain sympathetic. As he leaves the building, he notices Ms B standing nearby, and avoids her. The next day, Dr A tries to discuss the situation with a more senior doctor, Dr E, who tells him this sort of thing 'is quite common and will just blow over'.

- What else might Dr E have advised?

Dr A asks the receptionist not to book Ms B for him. Nonetheless, within a week another such appointment is booked, at which Ms B demands to know why Dr A seems to be avoiding her.

- What is happening with the receptionist?
- What might Dr A do now, and what might he be feeling?
- What about Ms B's feelings and actions?

Dr A realises he is 'out of his depth' and his sleep is becoming disturbed. He resolves to talk the issues through with both a trusted friend and his previous trainer and mentor. They help him conclude that he should have a discussion with his medical defence association and try to organise a regular practice-based continuous professional development session on 'difficult issues'.

The primary responsibility always lies with the doctor to keep the relationship professional.

Are there risky institutions?

While abuse of patients by doctors is highlighted here, the context is usually of a powerful individual in a collusive system. This could as easily be a nurse, a manager or another professional, even a member of the clergy. Scandals continue to emerge about whole institutions; for example, a 2011 TV programme about the Winterbourne View Care Home revealed widespread physical and psychological abuse of the learning-disabled patients. Characteristically, such institutions are secretive, isolated and have a strong 'us and them' internal culture. The residents or patients have little voice or power and complaints are ignored. Visitors, including doctors, may be shown a very limited view.

When is a patient not a patient?

A doctor takes up a practice on an island with a limited community, all of whom are his or her potential patients. Is he or she to have no relationships? What if a locum doctor sees a patient only once and there is mutual attraction? The GMC now provides further guidance on when someone may be regarded as no longer a patient and suggests taking into account the nature and length of the original professional relationship and seeking advice if in doubt. However:

> You must not pursue a sexual relationship with a former patient, where at the time of the professional relationship the patient was vulnerable, for example because of mental health problems, or because of their lack of maturity (General Medical Council, 2013).

The Royal College of Psychiatrists recommends against the forming of a sexual relationship with a former patient under any circumstances.

Your role as a witness

Doctors hold a trusted and privileged position. It can be difficult to raise concerns against powerful, charismatic people. In the past, one of the GMC's primary aims seemed to be to prevent one doctor from speaking ill of another. Now, however, there is a clear duty to 'express concern', especially on behalf of vulnerable patients and members staff. But to whom, and how? 'Whistle blowing' can still damage careers and cause a doctor to be labelled a troublemaker, so be prepared:

- Take advantage of any relevant training courses or workshops (e.g. on ethics or 'dealing with difficult colleagues').
- Organise local discussions, perhaps multidisciplinary (e.g. on the use of chaperones, when 'intimate examinations' are required or consent).
- Familiarise yourself with the local guidance on whistle blowing (which may be more about not reporting to the press than improving patient safety).
- Be ready to listen to patient complaints and find out how they can pursue them.

- Join a medical defence organisation: read its information and ask advice.
- Identify trusted seniors to ask for advice.
- It is best not to act alone, so keep colleagues onside.
- Documentation can be helpful.

Further reading

Celenza, A. & Gabbard, G.O. (2007) Analysts who commit sexual boundary violation: a lost cause? *FOCUS*, **5**, 483–492.

Council for Healthcare Regulatory Excellence (2008) Clear sexual boundaries between healthcare professionals and patients: responsibilities of healthcare professionals, http://www.professionalstandards.org.uk/docs /psa-library/responsibilities-of-healthcare-professionals---clear-sexual -boundaries.pdf?sfvrsn=0 (last accessed 12 February 2014).

Department of Health (2004) Committee of Inquiry – independent investigation into how the NHS handled allegations about the conduct of Clifford Ayling, http://webarchive.nationalarchives.gov.uk/20130107105354 /http://www.dh.gov.uk/en/Publicationsandstatistics/Publications /PublicationsPolicyAndGuidance/DH_4088996 (last accessed 12 February 2014).

Department of Health (2005) The Kerr/Haslam Inquiry, http://www.official -documents.gov.uk/document/cm66/6640/6640.asp (last accessed 12 February 2014).

Department of Health (2007) *Safeguarding Patients: The Government's Response to the Recommendations of the Shipman Inquiry's Fifth Report and to the Recommendations of the Ayling, Neale and Kerr/Haslam Inquiries.* Department of Health, London.

General Medical Council (2012) Raising and acting on concerns about patient safety, http://www.gmc-uk.org/guidance/ethical_guidance /raising_concerns.asp (last accessed 12 February 2014).

General Medical Council (2013) Maintaining a professional boundary between you and your patient, http://www.gmc-uk.org/guidance /ethical_guidance/21170.asp (last accessed 12 February 2014).

Gutheil, T.G. & Brodsky, A. (2008) *Preventing Boundary Violations in Clinical Practice.* Guilford Press, New York.

Subotsky, F., Bewley, S. & Crowe, M. (2010) *Abuse of the Doctor–Patient Relationship.* RCPsych, London.

Web sites

The Clinic for Boundaries Studies, www.professionalboundaries.org.uk (last accessed 12 February 2014).

Public Concern at Work (for whistle blowing advice), www.pcaw.org.uk (last accessed 12 February 2014).

Whistleblowing Helpline (for NHS and social care), www.wbhelpline.org.uk (last accessed 12 February 2014).

CHAPTER 25

Moving Forward: Developing Care Pathways within the Health Service

Loraine J. Bacchus

Department of Global Health and Development, Gender Violence and Health Centre, London School of Hygiene & Tropical Medicine, UK

> **OVERVIEW**
>
> - Primary and maternity health care provide favourable conditions in which to develop domestic violence interventions
> - These interventions include training and awareness raising, proactive identification of women affected by abuse and referral to support services
> - Partnership working includes voluntary and statutory organisations that support women and children affected by domestic violence, safeguarding leads, clinical champions and committed leaders in the health service
> - Key steps include training, guidelines, safe documentation, audits and research

Background

Primary and maternity health care are particularly favourable settings in which to offer proactive identification of women affected by domestic violence and referral pathways to support services. Health practitioners within these settings have opportunities to detect and deal with injuries and symptoms related to domestic violence and can create a confidential and safe space in which to ask sensitive questions. There is potential for offering longer consultations and continuity of care and for developing a patient–provider relationship and a philosophy of care that promotes shared decision making and recognises the social aspects of health. This chapter is designed to help health practitioners think about the types of intervention feasible within their health care setting, and strategies for successful implementation.

Committed leadership within the health care setting

Interventions require endorsement from senior clinicians and managers to help create and foster a 'domestic violence aware' culture. They also have an important function in endorsing change, such as the introduction of domestic violence clinical guidelines

and training, and in identifying resources (e.g. staff, time and finances) so as to ensure the sustainability of any intervention. If there is no clinical lead for domestic violence, it is possible to incorporate the issue within an existing NHS lead role, such as safeguarding children or vulnerable adults. Even as a junior doctor, you can champion the issue in the department.

Awareness raising and sensitisation of health practitioners

This is required in identifying and supporting women affected by domestic violence and before delivering any training programme. Sensitisation activities include: giving presentations or lectures on the prevalence and health impact of domestic violence and national policy recommendations surrounding it; inviting representatives from domestic violence specialist organisations to give talks; and discussing actual case studies of domestic violence in clinical meetings. Interested doctors and midwives can be part of this process; such clinicians are sometimes referred to as 'clinical champions' for domestic violence. You can be part of this process even as a junior in training. It is good practice for clinical champions to be formally recognised and supported in their activities by managers. They might undertake a literature search or a brief waiting room survey on domestic violence to collate local data on the extent of the problem and, as identified experts, they are also the liaison with local multi-agency domestic violence fora and crime and disorder-reduction partnerships. Observing or attending meetings can be a useful training opportunity for a junior doctor.

Clinical guidelines

These provide clear guidance on interventions, maintain staff and patient safety, and deal with confidentiality and responsible information sharing. Guidelines might include asking questions about domestic violence of all women versus just those with risk markers. They ought to consider a safe system for documenting domestic violence in the patient record (whether/when the patient was asked about domestic violence, her response and any referral offered). This might be via printed notes, a 'stamp' or a pro forma. Particular care has to be taken with handheld notes or where information might not be 'safe' or confidential. Regular audits with feedback

---

ABC of Domestic and Sexual Violence, First Edition.
Edited by Susan Bewley and Jan Welch.
© 2014 John Wiley & Sons, Ltd. Published 2014 by John Wiley & Sons, Ltd.

can be performed to motivate staff, implement change and monitor practice. Department of Health (2005) and National Institute for Health and Care and Excellence (2014) guidelines can be adapted to the local context. Make links with academics with expertise on gender violence and health in order to jointly apply for funding to conduct research. A junior might adapt a guideline, customise it locally and pilot, audit and implement it.

Develop a rolling programme of domestic violence training

Many specialist domestic violence services offer training. Training, preferably mandatory, should take place within the health care setting. It should be delivered regularly in order to capture new and rotating staff. Experiential evidence shows that training programmes are best designed collaboratively between specialist domestic violence organisations and clinicians, who can comment on how best to introduce enquiry or documentation practices into their routine clinical care.

Case studies and research used in training should be relevant to the health care setting and trainers should take into consideration the practitioners' clinical environment, roles and responsibilities. Health practitioners can provide examples of actual domestic violence cases for discussion in the training. Pre-training assessments are recommended, as different members of staff will have different skills, knowledge and experience, and will require different levels of training. Learners can be motivated by being informed that they will become more skilled practitioners, equipped to ask deeper questions about 'what's going on at home' – particularly with those patients who do not attend, do not comply, have complex needs or discharge themselves against advice. They will learn that these are not 'difficult patients', but patients with difficult problems.

Training has to be department-wide in order to ensure competence of the whole team. Using clinicians as co-trainers helps to gain acceptance, as they model good practice and can legitimately deal with staff resistance. Consider incentive schemes such as linking the training to continuing professional development. Reinforcement training activities such as sharing good practice in dealing with domestic violence cases and updates from trainers are important to sustaining change.

Identifying and developing appropriate referral pathways

Appropriate pathways for women affected by domestic violence depend upon what services and resources are available locally. Whether health practitioners are proactively identifying domestic violence or not, they must establish links with local organisations to which they can refer women and children affected by abuse.

A number of models have been tested in primary and maternity care settings in Europe (see Boxes 25.1, 25.2 and 25.3). Other examples that might be adapted can be found in a recent scoping study, which identified best practice recommendations for implementing and sustaining interventions (Bacchus *et al.*, 2012). Finally, a recent systematic review provides the international evidence for interventions in health care settings. This needs to be referenced as

Feder et al. 2009 which is in the reference list so that people know how to access it

Box 25.1 **MOZAIC Women's Wellbeing Project**

This is a partnership in the UK between an NHS hospital trust and a voluntary-sector women's organisation. An 'in reach' approach is utilised whereby independent domestic violence advisors (IDVAs) based in the hospital provide direct support to women (see Chapters 8 and 9). They train health professionals and strengthen links with other organisations in the community. This model has been formally evaluated and changes have been found in clinical practice, including an increase in routine enquiry for domestic violence.

Box 25.2 **Mentor mothers (MeMoSA)**

In the Netherlands, a trial is currently being undertaken in GP settings in Nijmegen, with mentor mothers supporting women with young children. Women meet with a mentor mother once or twice a week for 4 months to focus on: cessation/reduction of violence, children who witness violence, management of depressive complaints and improvement of women's social networks to reduce isolation. Mentor mothers receive training and support from domestic violence specialists.

Box 25.3 **Identification and Referral to Improve Safety (IRIS) trial**

In GP settings in the UK, the IRIS trial demonstrates the effectiveness of a brief intervention consisting of training for GPs, clinical enquiry for domestic violence based on certain diagnoses and a simple referral pathway to a named advocate from a specialist domestic violence organisation. The advocate is also responsible for training GPs ensuring that the intervention is embedded within a close partnership with the domestic violence organisation.

Twenty-four practices received the intervention and twenty-four did not. Twelve months after training there was a significant increase in referral to advocacy in the intervention group. Each intervention practice also had a clinical champion, a doctor or nurse who was invited to attend further training to ensure that the work was integrated into the practice.

Listen to survivors

It is important to listen to those who use these domestic violence services. Feedback on their views and experiences of the service and how it might be developed in the future can be elicited through formal research and evaluation, or by setting up a survivors' group that meets regularly.

Evaluation and monitoring

Evaluation and monitoring of the intervention is necessary to demonstrate to staff (and potential funders) the benefit to patients. At the very least, include a safe coding system in the patient

Table 25.1 Challenges and opportunities.

Challenges	Opportunities
Convincing health practitioners that domestic violence is a health issue	Establish links with local voluntary and statutory organisations through your local multi-agency domestic violence forum Invite a local specialist domestic violence organisation to present at a meeting Refer to national policy and guidance and discuss cases of domestic violence at clinical meetings Conduct an anonymous domestic violence survey in the clinic
Initiating changes in clinical practice	Identify, or become, a clinical champion with an interest in domestic violence Identify and make links with the child and adult safeguarding leads in the local hospital Trust or health and wellbeing board Check that the human resources department has policies to support staff affected by domestic violence Have domestic violence posters and leaflets on display at the clinic
Developing tailored domestic violence training	Find a local specialist domestic violence organisation that offers training and develop training that is specific to your health context Use health practitioners as co-trainers
Motivating health professionals to attend training	Make domestic violence training mandatory; link to continuing professional development and include in child and adult safeguarding training Offer training during and outside of normal working hours
Evaluating and monitoring changes in practice	Develop clinical guidelines that include guidance on how to ask questions about domestic violence safely Be clear about where and how to document abuse safely and where to refer women Include a domestic violence coding scheme in the patient record and conduct regular audits to feed back Explore funding for health service research with academics
Sustaining the intervention	Ensure clinical champions and staff at a senior and strategic level are involved at all stages of development of the intervention Keep domestic violence on the agenda at clinical and academic meetings Ensure a rolling programme of ongoing training to capture new staff and maintain a 'domestic violence aware' culture Use short reinforcement training activities (e.g. actual case studies and discussion, audits of patient records and results from research) to share and sustain good practice Find funding to commission for advocacy services

records that indicates whether or not a patient has been asked about domestic violence, their response and any referrals. Conduct regular audits of the domestic violence code, which can be presented at clinical meetings and used in any reinforcement training. Identify academic experts in the field of gender violence and health with whom you can apply for funding to develop and conduct research on an intervention in your health care setting.

Challenges and opportunities

Challenges and opportunities going forward are listed in Table 25.1.

Further reading

Bacchus, L.J., Aston, G., Torres Vitolas, C., Jordan, P. & Murray, S.F. (2007) *A Theory-Based Evaluation of a Multi-Agency Domestic Violence Service Based in Maternity and Genitourinary Medicine Services at Guy's & St. Thomas' NHS Foundation Trust.* King's College London, London, http://gender violence.lshtm.ac.uk/files/Bacchus-et-al-2007-full-report-MOZAIC1.pdf (last accessed 12 February 2014).

Bacchus, L., Bewley, S., Aston, G., Torres Vitolas, C., Jordan, P. & Murray, S.F. (2010) Evaluation of a UK domestic violence intervention in maternity and sexual health services. *Reproductive Health Matters*, **18**, 147–157.

Bacchus, L.J., Fernandez, C., Hellbernd, H., Lo Fo Wong, S., Pas, L., Perttu, S., Savola, T., Bewley, S. & Otasevic, S. (2012) *Health Sector Responses To Domestic Violence: Promising Intervention Models in Primary and Maternity Health Care Settings in Europe.* London School of Hygiene & Tropical Medicine, London, http://diverhse.eu/project-outputs/ (last accessed 12 February 2014).

Department of Health (2005) *Responding to Domestic Abuse: A Handbook for Health Professionals.* Department of Health, London, http://webarchive .nationalarchives.gov.uk/20130107105354/http://www.dh.gov.uk/en /Publicationsandstatistics/Publications/PublicationsPolicyAndGuidance /DH_4126161 (last accessed 12 February 2014).

Feder, G., Ramsay, J., Dunne, D., Rose, M., Arsene, C., Norman, R., Kuntze, S., Spencer, A., Bacchus, L., Hague, G., Warburton, A. & Taket, A. (2009) How far does screening women for domestic (partner) violence in different health-care settings meet criteria for a screening programme? Systematic reviews of nine UK National Screening Committee criteria. *Health Technology Assessment*, **13**, 1–136, http://www.hta.ac.uk/1501 (last accessed 12 February 2014).

Feder, G., Davies, R.A., Baird, K., Dunne, D., Eldridge, S., Griffiths, C., Gregory, A., Howell, A., Johnson, M., Ramsay, J., Rutterford, C. & Sharp, D. (2011) Identification and Referral to Improve Safety (IRIS) of women experiencing domestic violence with a primary care training and support programme: a cluster randomised controlled trial. *Lancet*, **378**, 1788–1795.

Loeffen, M.J.W., Lo Fo Wong, S., Wester, F.P.J.F., Laurant, M.G.H. & Lagro-Janssen, A.L.M. (2011) Implementing mentor mothers in family practice to support abused mothers: study protocol. *BMC Family Practice*, **12**, 113.

National Institute for Health and Care and Excellence (2014) Domestic violence and abuse – identification and prevention, http://guidance.nice.org .uk/PHG/44 (last accessed 12 February 2014).

Torres Vitolas, C., Bacchus, L. & Aston, G. (2010) A comparison of the training needs of maternity and sexual health professionals in a London teaching hospital with regards to routine enquiry for domestic abuse. *Public Health*, **124**, 472–478.

CHAPTER 26

Moving Forward: Pursuing a Career and Implementing Better Services

Maureen Dalton

SARC Commissioning South West, UK

> **OVERVIEW**
> - All doctors now have to have basic competence from registration
> - More is required for child safeguarding
> - Further training and specialisation are available
> - Audits, teaching and research contribute to continuous quality improvement

Domestic abuse

From the outset of your career, you need to be aware of the needs of victims of domestic abuse and sexual assault. During your career you will see many victims of domestic abuse, even if they are not immediately apparent. It will be a good core skill to have a solid understanding of the issues. These are included in the new foundation programme for qualifying doctors, which emphasises the competences needed in the 'good clinical care' section (see Box 26.1).

Box 26.1 **Foundation years competency**

Demonstrates the ability to identify, refer to and participate in both medical assessment and care planning in cases where the interests of a child or vulnerable adult, including those with learning difficulties or who are a potential victim of abuse, need safeguarding. Demonstrates an awareness of the potential for physical, psychological and sexual abuse of patients, and manages such cases in a similar way to the safeguarding of children and vulnerable adults.

If it was not well covered during undergraduate training, it is a good idea to consider a domestic abuse course early on. These are not run by many hospital trusts but they may be available from your local domestic abuse forum. There are various e-learning packages on the subject, including the Royal College of General Practitioners course, which is free to other health practitioners and is a good first step.

The National Institute for Health and Care and Excellence has recently developed public health guidelines, published in 2014. The Department of Health Taskforce on tackling Violence against Women and Children has recommended that domestic abuse features in both undergraduate and postgraduate syllabuses and be part of routine continuing professional development. Many royal colleges are considering how to implement this.

Child safeguarding

An intercollegiate document sets out the safeguarding competences (i.e. the knowledge, skills, attitudes and values required) for safe and effective practice by health workers (Royal College of Paediatrics and Child Health, 2010). All doctors need to have level 2 training (see Box 26.2) and doctors who see children as a significant part of their work (i.e. most doctors) must be trained to level 3. Some additional competences are required for certain specialities, such as forensic physicians, paediatricians and child and adolescent psychiatrists. Levels 4–6 are set for specialists and experts in safeguarding.

Box 26.2 **Child safeguarding training**

- **Level 1:** All clinical and nonclinical staff.
- **Level 2:** All clinical staff with any contact with children.
- **Level 3:** All clinical staff working with children.
- **Levels 4–6:** Specialist roles.

Most hospital trusts run frequent level 1 and 2 child protection courses or have easily accessible e-learning packages.

Sexual assault

The care of victims of sexual assault is less well covered in medical training, yet poor care increases the workload of the NHS. It has been estimated that 50% of patients in the mental health services have been a victim of sexual assault, and the percentage in acute psychiatric hospitals is even higher. The Home Office, together with The Havens, has developed a useful e-learning package comprising two modules: 'care of a victim' and 'evidence' (www.careandevidence.org). It also has guidance on such aspects

---

ABC of Domestic and Sexual Violence, First Edition.
Edited by Susan Bewley and Jan Welch.
© 2014 John Wiley & Sons, Ltd. Published 2014 by John Wiley & Sons, Ltd.

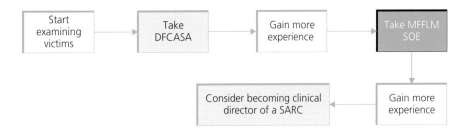

Figure 26.1 Career pathway and considerations. DFCASA, Diploma in Forensic and Clinical Aspects of Sexual Assault; MFFLM, Member of the Faculty of Forensic and Legal Medicine; SOE, sexual offences examiner; SARC, sexual assault referral centre.

of care as who should be considered for HIV post-exposure prophylaxis following sexual exposure (PEPSE).

If you want to develop your care of victims of sexual assault further, there is now a fairly clear series of steps. The Diploma in Forensic and Clinical Aspects of Sexual Assault (DFCASA) has been developed with help from the Department of Health and is set at the basic level of competence required to examine a victim. It is designed to be suitable for both doctors and nurses.

The Faculty of Forensic and Legal Medicine (FFLM), part of the Royal College of Physicians, has a membership exam specifically for sexual offence examiners: the MFFLM (SOM). This is more advanced than the DFCASA and is only open to doctors. The FFLM is also developing modular credentialing, which if successful will allow a route on to the specialist register.

The Royal College of Obstetrics and Gynaecology has developed an Advanced Specialist Training module on Leadership in Domestic Violence and Sexual Assault Services.

These building blocks are now in place to allow you to become better trained in the issues of domestic and sexual abuse, to improve the general care of victims and to consider sexual offences medicine as a possible career route (see Figure 26.1).

At all stages of your career, you can proactively develop knowledge, skills and attitudes in line with General Medical Council requirements and so further contribute to the care of your patients who have experienced domestic and sexual violence (see Boxes 26.3, 26.4 and 26.5).

Box 26.3 How to improve your knowledge, skills, attitudes and curriculum vitae

- Learn more – both factual (see Further Reading and Box 26.4) and empathic (e.g. narratives in Box 26.5).
- Speak out and educate others.
- Perform an audit. This might relate to the knowledge of staff in your department of local sources of support for victims of domestic abuse/sexual assault or to their knowledge of what to do when a patient reveals they have been a recent victim of domestic abuse/sexual assault. If your department sees children, audit the knowledge staff have of the risk assessment tools for domestic and child abuse.
- Think about how to integrate this interest in your future career (e.g. in general practice or such specialties as forensic paediatrics, forensic psychiatry and forensic pathology). Try to talk to people working in these specialties in order to gain greater insight. Go to the appropriate college Web site to get a better view of the training requirements and number of potential vacancies in the specialty in which you wish to specialise. You may be able to

spend a day or two shadowing someone doing that job, as often what they are doing will be in a different area of the specialty to that in which you are exposed as a student. Remember that the TV versions of the post do not represent the reality!

- Consider volunteering or donating your time and money to charities (e.g. Women's Aid, Freedom from Torture) or to other campaigning organisations (e.g. Physicians for Human Rights, the White Ribbon Alliance).
- Do a sponsored marathon, cycle ride or other project to raise money for an appropriate charity. A CV that says, 'I have raised £5 000 for Women's Aid by running four marathons' looks better than one that says, 'I like to run in my spare time'.
- Consider offering peer education to medical students and foundation years covering domestic and sexual violence.
- If you have a second language, you may be able to give talks or help educate local groups from that ethnic community on the effects of domestic and sexual abuse and how they can find suitable resources or ask for help.

Box 26.4 Continuing professional development and learning resources

- British Association for Sexual Health and HIV (BASHH) & Federation of the Royal Colleges of Physicians, in partnership with DH e-Learning for Healthcare. E-learning module for HIV and sexual health, http://www.e-lfh.org.uk/projects/sexual-health-and-hiv/ (last accessed 12 February 2014).
- Care and Evidence Web site, www.careandevidence.org (last accessed 12 February 2014).
- Diploma in the Forensic and Clinical Aspects of Sexual Assault (DFCASA), http://www.apothecaries.org/examination/diploma-in-the-forensic-and-clinical-aspects-of-se/ (last accessed 12 February 2014).
- FGM National Clinical Group Web site, www.fgmnationalgroup.org (last accessed 12 February 2014).
- General Medical Council (no date) Duties of a doctor, http://www.gmc-uk.org/guidance/good_medical_practice/duties_of_a_doctor.asp (last accessed 12 February 2014).
- Royal College of General Practitioners (no date) Domestic violence e-learning package, http://elearning.rcgp.org.uk/login/index.php (last accessed 12 February 2014).
- Royal College of Paediatrics and Child Health (2010) Safeguarding children and young people (SGC), http://www.rcpch.ac.uk/safeguarding (last accessed 12 February 2014).
- Royal College of Physicians: Faculty of Forensic & Legal Medicine (no date) MFFLM examination, http://fflm.ac.uk/education/mfflmexam/ (last accessed 12 February 2014).

- Royal College of Obstetrics and Gynaecology (no date) ATSM: forensic gynaecology, http://www.rcog.org.uk/curriculum-module /atsm-forensic-gynaecology (last accessed 12 February 2014).
- Taskforce on the Health Aspects of Violence Against Women and Children (2010) *Responding to Violence against Women and Children – the Role of the NHS*, http://webarchive.national archives.gov.uk/20130107105354/http://www.dh.gov.uk/prod _consum_dh/groups/dh_digitalassets/@dh/@en/@ps/documents /digitalasset/dh_113824.pdf (last accessed 12 February 2014).

Box 26.5 Some books and films that may stimulate empathy, discussion and learning

The Color Purple by Alice Walker (1982 novel, 1985 film).
Sleeping with the Enemy by Nancy Price (1987 novel, 1991 film).
The Accused by Tom Topor (1988 film).
Waverley Place by Susan Brownmiller (1989 novel).
This Boy's Life by Tobias Wolff (1989 novel, 1993 film).
The Stranger Beside Me by Ann Rule (1980 book, 1995 film).
Push by Sapphire (1996 novel); adapted as *Precious* (2009 film).
The Woman Who Walked into Doors by Roddy Doyle (1996 novel).
It Could Have Been You by Merlyn Nuttall (1998).
The Perks of Being a Wallflower by Stephen Chbosky (1999 novel, 2012 film).
Lucky (1999) and *The Lovely Bones* (2002 novel, 2010 film) by Alice Sebold.
Enough by Nicholas Kazan (2002 film).
No Ordinary Man: A Life of George Carman by Dominic Carmen (2002 book).
Provoked by Carl Austin & Rahila Gupta (2006 film).
This Charming Man by Marian Keyes (2008 novel).

Conclusion

Responding to domestic and sexual violence can be a small part of any doctor's job, a large part of some doctors' jobs in a variety of specialities or a full-time job in a few specialties. Whatever specialty you end up in, do keep listening and learning from patients.

Further reading

Dalton, M. (eds) (2013) *Forensic Gynaecology*. RCOG Press.

Dalton, M. (eds) (2013) *Best Practice & Research*. Clinical Obstetrics & Gynaecology Volume **27**, Issue 1. Elsevier.

Office of the Children's Commissioner (no date) Inquiry into child sexual exploitation in gangs and groups (CSEGG), http://www.childrens commissioner.gov.uk/info/csegg1 (last accessed 12 February 2014).

Royal College of Paediatrics and Child Health (2010) Safeguarding children and young people (SGC), http://www.rcpch.ac.uk/safeguarding (last accessed 12 February 2014).

Taskforce on the Health Aspects of Violence Against Women and Children (2010) *Responding to Violence against Women and Children – The Role of the NHS*, http://webarchive.nationalarchives.gov.uk/20130107105354 /http://www.dh.gov.uk/prod_consum_dh/groups/dh_digitalassets/@dh /@en/@ps/documents/digitalasset/dh_113824.pdf (last accessed 12 February 2014).

White, C. (2010) *Sexual Assault: A Forensic Clinician's Practice Guide*. St Mary's Sexual Assault Referral Centre.

World Bank (no date) Gender-based violence, health and the role of the health sector, http://web.worldbank.org/WBSITE/EXTERNAL/TOPICS /EXTHEALTHNUTRITIONANDPOPULATION/EXTPHAAG/0,,content MDK:22421973~pagePK:64229817~piPK:64229743~theSitePK: 672263,00.html (last accessed 12 February 2014).

World Health Organization (no date) Gender-based violence, http://www.who .int/gender/violence/gbv/en/index.html (last accessed 12 February 2014).

APPENDIX A

Useful Resources

Key national support services

National Domestic Violence Helpline, www.nationaldomesticviolence helpline.org.uk (last accessed 12 February 2014). Women can be referred to the 24 hour freephone (run in partnership between Women's Aid and Refuge): 0808 2000 247.

NHS Choices Website, www.nhs.uk (last accessed 12 February 2014). Offers help after sexual assault and rape (http://www.nhs.uk/Livewell /Sexualhealth/Pages/Sexualassault.aspx) and provides a postcode search for sexual violence services and SARCs (http://www.nhs.uk/Service-Search/Rape-and-sexual-assault-referral-centres/LocationSearch/364).

Men's Advice Line, 0808 801 0327, www.mensadviceline.org.uk (last accessed 12 February 2014). For men who experience domestic violence or abuse.

Rape Crisis Centres, 0808 802 99 99, www.rapecrisis.org.uk (last accessed 12 February 2014).

Samaritans, 08457 90 90 90 (24 hours a day), www.samaritans.org (last accessed 12 February 2014).

UK Government Forced Marriage Unit, 0207 008 0151, http://www.gov.uk /forced-marriage. Works across the world dealing with cases of forced marriage.

Women's Aid, www.womensaid.org.uk (last accessed 12 February 2014). Local support services throughout the UK are listed on the Women's Aid Web site.

Specialist services, charities, campaigning and self-help groups

Action on Elder Abuse, www.elderabuse.org.uk (last accessed 12 February 2014).

Ashiana, www.ashiana.org.uk (last accessed 12 February 2014). A charitable organisation based in London that helps women from the Asian, Turkish and Iranian communities. Ashiana's services include refuge accommodation and support for young women at risk of/fleeing from forced marriage.

Broken Rainbow, www.broken-rainbow.org.uk (last accessed 12 February 2014). Advice for lesbian, gay, bisexual and transgender patients.

Daughters of Eve, www.dofeve.org (last accessed 12 February 2014). A non-profit organisation that works to protect girls and young women who are at risk from female genital mutilation.

Eaves Poppy Project, www.eavesforwomen.org.uk (last accessed 12 February 2014). Supports trafficked women or women wanting to escape prostitution.

Forward, www.forwarduk.org (last accessed 12 February 2014). An African diaspora women-led UK-registered campaign and support charity dedicated to advancing and safeguarding the sexual and reproductive health and rights of African girls and women.

Freedom Charity, www.freedomcharity.org.uk (last accessed 12 February 2014). Concerned with children and young people who are vulnerable to violent crimes, dishonour-based violence and forced marriages. Offers a free iPhone app that can provide help and assistance.

Human Trafficking Foundation, www.humantraffickingfoundation.org (last accessed 12 February 2014).

Imkaan, imkaan.org.uk (last accessed 12 February 2014). An organisation dedicated to challenging violence against black, minority ethnic and refugee women and children.

Iranian & Kurdish Women's Rights Organisation (IKWRO), 0207 920 6460, www.ikwro.org.uk (last accessed 12 February 2014). Provides advice and support to Middle Eastern women and girls living in the UK who face 'honour'-based violence, domestic abuse, forced marriage or female genital mutilation.

nia, www.niaendingviolence.org.uk (last accessed 12 February 2014). Works with girls and gangs and helps prevent sexual violence and exploitation. The Safe Choices programme works with young women who experience a number of risk factors in relation to gang culture.

Karma Nirvana, www.karmanirvana.org.uk (last accessed 12 February 2014). Runs an Honour Network Helpline: 08005 999 247.

Platform51 (previously YWCA), platform51.org (last accessed 12 February 2014). Helps young women in trouble or who have been trafficked women.

Positively UK, positivelyuk.org (last accessed 12 February 2014). A national charity that can provide peer support that campaigns for the rights of people living with HIV.

Refuge, www.refuge.org.uk (last accessed 12 February 2014). Supports women and children through refuges, independent advocacy, community outreach and culturally specific services.

Respect, 0808 802 4040, www.respect.uk.net (last accessed 12 February 2014). For domestic violence perpetrators and professionals who would like further information on services for those using violence/abuse in their intimate partner relationships.

Salvation Army, www.salvationarmy.org.uk (last accessed 12 February 2014). Supports trafficked women and women wanting to escape prostitution.

Solace Women's Aid, www.solacewomensaid.org (last accessed 12 February 2014).

ABC of Domestic and Sexual Violence, First Edition.
Edited by Susan Bewley and Jan Welch.
© 2014 John Wiley & Sons, Ltd. Published 2014 by John Wiley & Sons, Ltd.

Southall Black Sisters, www.southallblacksisters.org.uk (last accessed 12 February 2014). A not-for-profit organisation set up to meet the needs of black (Asian and African-Caribbean) and minority ethnic women.

Survivors UK, www.survivorsuk.org (last accessed 12 February 2014). A self-help organisation that supports men who have experienced sexual assault and rape as children or adults.

Victim Support, www.victimsupport.org.uk (last accessed 12 February 2014). The national charity for victims of crime.

Women & Girls Network, www.wgn.org.uk (last accessed 12 February 2014). Offers counselling and support for women who have experienced gendered violence.

CAADA-DASH Risk Identification Checklist

CAADA-DASH Risk Identification Checklist (RIC)[i] for MARAC Agencies

Aim of the form:

- To help front line practitioners identify high risk cases of domestic abuse, stalking and 'honour'-based violence.
- To decide which cases should be referred to MARAC and what other support might be required. A completed form becomes an active record that can be referred to in future for case management.
- To offer a common tool to agencies that are part of the MARAC[1] process and provide a shared understanding of risk in relation to domestic abuse, stalking and 'honour'-based violence.
- To enable agencies to make defensible decisions based on the evidence from extensive research of cases, including domestic homicides and 'near misses', which underpins most recognised models of risk assessment.

How to use the form:

Before completing the form for the first time we recommend that you read the full practice guidance and Frequently Asked Questions and Answers[2]. These can be downloaded from http://www.caada.org.uk/marac/RIC_for_MARAC.html. Risk is dynamic and can change very quickly. It is good practice to review the checklist after a new incident.

Recommended Referral Criteria to MARAC

1. **Professional judgement:** if a professional has serious concerns about a victim's situation, they should refer the case to MARAC. There will be occasions where the particular context of a case gives rise to serious concerns even if the victim has been unable to disclose the information that might highlight their risk more clearly. *This could reflect extreme levels of fear, cultural barriers to disclosure, immigration issues or language barriers particularly in cases of 'honour'-based violence.* This judgement would be based on the professional's experience and/or the victim's perception of their risk even if they do not meet criteria 2 and/or 3 below.

2. **'Visible High Risk':** the number of 'ticks' on this checklist. If you have ticked 14 or more 'yes' boxes the case would normally meet the MARAC referral criteria.

3. **Potential Escalation:** the number of police callouts to the victim as a result of domestic violence in the past 12 months. This criterion can be used to identify cases where there is not a positive identification of a majority of the risk factors on the list, but where abuse appears to be escalating and where it is appropriate to assess the situation more fully by sharing information at MARAC. It is common practice to start with 3 or more police callouts in a 12 month period but this will need to be reviewed depending on your local volume and your level of police reporting.

Please pay particular attention to a practitioner's professional judgement in all cases. The results from a checklist are not a definitive assessment of risk. They should provide you with a structure to inform your judgement and act as prompts to further questioning, analysis and risk management whether via a MARAC or in another way.

The responsibility for identifying your local referral threshold rests with your local MARAC.

What this form is not:

This form will provide valuable information about the risks that children are living with but it is not a full risk assessment for children. The presence of children increases the wider risks of domestic violence and step children are particularly at risk. If risk towards children is highlighted you should consider what referral you need to make to obtain a full assessment of the children's situation.

---

[1] For further information about MARAC please refer to the 10 Principles of an Effective MARAC:
http://www.caada.org.uk/marac/10_Principles_Oct_2011_full.doc

[2] For enquiries about training in the use of the form, please email training@caada.org.uk or call 0117 317 8750.

Web www.caada.org.uk E-mail marac@caada.org.uk Tel 0117 317 8750

ABC of Domestic and Sexual Violence, First Edition.
Edited by Susan Bewley and Jan Welch.
© 2014 John Wiley & Sons, Ltd. Published 2014 by John Wiley & Sons, Ltd.

Name of victim: **Date:** **Restricted when completed**

CAADA-DASH Risk Identification Checklist for use by IDVAs and other non-police agencies[3] for identification of risks when domestic abuse, 'honour'-based violence and/or stalking are disclosed

Please explain that the purpose of asking these questions is for the safety and protection of the individual concerned. Tick the box if the factor is present ☑. Please use the comment box at the end of the form to expand on any answer. It is assumed that your main source of information is the victim. If this is not the case please indicate in the right hand column	Yes (tick)	No	Don't Know	State source of info if not the victim e.g. police officer
1. Has the current incident resulted in injury? (Please state what and whether this is the first injury.)	☐	☐	☐	
2. Are you very frightened? Comment:	☐	☐	☐	
3. What are you afraid of? Is it further injury or violence? (Please give an indication of what you think (name of abuser(s)...) might do and to whom, including children). Comment:	☐	☐	☐	
4. Do you feel isolated from family/friends i.e. does (name of abuser(s) ....) try to stop you from seeing friends/family/doctor or others? Comment:	☐	☐	☐	
5. Are you feeling depressed or having suicidal thoughts?	☐	☐	☐	
6. Have you separated or tried to separate from (name of abuser(s)...,) within the past year?	☐	☐	☐	
7. Is there conflict over child contact?	☐	☐	☐	
8. Does (......) constantly text, call, contact, follow, stalk or harass you? (Please expand to identify what and whether you believe that this is done deliberately to intimidate you? Consider the context and behaviour of what is being done.)	☐	☐	☐	
9. Are you pregnant or have you recently had a baby (within the last 18 months)?	☐	☐	☐	
10. Is the abuse happening more often?	☐	☐	☐	
11. Is the abuse getting worse?	☐	☐	☐	
12. Does (......) try to control everything you do and/or are they excessively jealous? (In terms of relationships, who you see, being 'policed at home', telling you what to wear for example. Consider 'honour'-based violence and specify behaviour.)	☐	☐	☐	

[3] Note: This checklist is consistent with the ACPO endorsed risk assessment model DASH 2009 for the police service.

Web www.caada.org.uk E-mail marac@caada.org.uk Tel 0117 317 8750
© CAADA 2012. Please acknowledge CAADA when reprinting. Registered charity number 1106864

Name of victim: **Date:** **Restricted when completed**

Tick box if factor is present. Please use the comment box at the end of the form to expand on any answer.	Yes (tick)	No	Don't Know	State source of info if not the victim
13. Has (........) ever used weapons or objects to hurt you?	☐	☐	☐	
14. Has (........) ever threatened to kill you or someone else and you believed them? (If yes, tick who.) You ☐ Children ☐ Other (please specify) ☐	☐	☐	☐	
15. Has (.........) ever attempted to strangle/choke/suffocate/drown you?	☐	☐	☐	
16. Does (........) do or say things of a sexual nature that make you feel bad or that physically hurt you or someone else? (If someone else, specify who.)	☐	☐	☐	
17. Is there any other person who has threatened you or who you are afraid of? (If yes, please specify whom and why. Consider extended family if HBV.)	☐	☐	☐	
18. Do you know if (..........) has hurt anyone else? (Please specify whom including the children, siblings or elderly relatives. Consider HBV.) Children ☐ Another family member ☐ Someone from a previous relationship ☐ Other (please specify) ☐	☐	☐	☐	
19. Has (..........) ever mistreated an animal or the family pet?	☐	☐	☐	
20. Are there any financial issues? For example, are you dependent on (.....) for money/have they recently lost their job/other financial issues?	☐	☐	☐	
21. Has (........) had problems in the past year with drugs (prescription or other), alcohol or mental health leading to problems in leading a normal life? (If yes, please specify which and give relevant details if known.) Drugs ☐ Alcohol ☐ Mental Health ☐	☐	☐	☐	
22. Has (......) ever threatened or attempted suicide?	☐	☐	☐	
23. Has (.........) ever broken bail/an injunction and/or formal agreement for when they can see you and/or the children? (You may wish to consider this in relation to an ex-partner of the perpetrator if relevant.) Bail conditions ☐ Non Molestation/Occupation Order ☐ Child Contact arrangements ☐ Forced Marriage Protection Order ☐ Other ☐	☐	☐	☐	
24. Do you know if (........) has ever been in trouble with the police or has a criminal history? (If yes, please specify.) DV ☐ Sexual violence ☐ Other violence ☐ Other ☐	☐	☐	☐	
Total 'yes' responses				

Web www.caada.org.uk E-mail marac@caada.org.uk Tel 0117 317 8750
© CAADA 2012. Please acknowledge CAADA when reprinting. Registered charity number 1106864

Name of victim: **Date:**   **Restricted when completed**

For consideration by professional: Is there any other relevant information (from victim or professional) which may increase risk levels? Consider victim's situation in relation to disability, substance misuse, mental health issues, cultural/language barriers, 'honour'- based systems, geographic isolation and minimisation. Are they willing to engage with your service? Describe: Consider abuser's occupation/interests - could this give them unique access to weapons? Describe:
What are the victim's greatest priorities to address their safety?
Do you believe that there are reasonable grounds for referring this case to MARAC? Yes / No If yes, have you made a referral? Yes/No **Signed:**   **Date:**
Do you believe that there are risks facing the children in the family? Yes / No If yes, please confirm if you have made a referral to safeguard the children: Yes / No Date referral made ……………………………………….
Signed: **Date:** **Name:**

Practitioner's Notes

---

[i] This checklist reflects work undertaken by CAADA in partnership with Laura Richards, Consultant Violence Adviser to ACPO. We would like to thank Advance, Blackburn with Darwen Women's Aid and Berkshire East Family Safety Unit and all the partners of the Blackpool MARAC for their contribution in piloting the revised checklist without which we could not have amended the original CAADA risk identification checklist. We are very grateful to Elizabeth Hall of Cafcass and Neil Blacklock of Respect for their advice and encouragement and for the expert input we received from Jan Pickles, Dr Amanda Robinson and Jasvinder Sanghera.

Web www.caada.org.uk E-mail marac@caada.org.uk Tel 0117 317 8750

Index

ABC of Pain

Lesley A. Colvin & Marie Fallon
Western General Hospital, Edinburgh; University of Edinburgh

Pain is a common presentation and this brand new title focuses on the pain management issues most often encountered in primary care. *ABC of Pain*:

- Covers all the chronic pain presentations in primary care right through to tertiary and palliative care and includes guidance on pain management in special groups such as pregnancy, children, the elderly and the terminally ill
- Includes new findings on the effectiveness of interventions and the progression to acute pain and appropriate pharmacological management
- Features pain assessment, epidemiology and the evidence base in a truly comprehensive reference
- Provides a global perspective with an international list of expert contributors

JUNE 2012 | 9781405176217 | 128 PAGES | £24.99/US$44.95/€32.90/AU$47.95

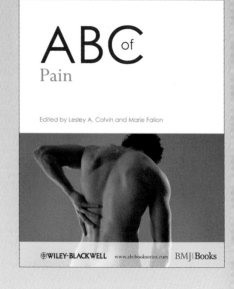

ABC of Urology

3RD EDITION

Chris Dawson & Janine Nethercliffe
Fitzwilliam Hospital, Peterborough; Edith Cavell Hospital, Peterborough

Urological conditions are common, accounting for up to one third of all surgical admissions to hospital. Outside of hospital care urological problems are a common reason for patients needing to see their GP.

- *ABC of Urology, 3rd Edition* provides a comprehensive overview of urology
- Focuses on the diagnosis and management of the most common urological conditions
- Features 4 additional chapters: improved coverage of renal and testis cancer in separate chapters and new chapters on management of haematuria, laparoscopy, trauma and new urological advances
- Ideal for GPs and trainee GPs, and is useful for junior doctors undergoing surgical training, while medical students and nurses undertaking a urological placement as part of their training programme will find this edition indispensable

MARCH 2012 | 9780470657171 | 88 PAGES | £23.99/US$37.95/€30.90/AU$47.95

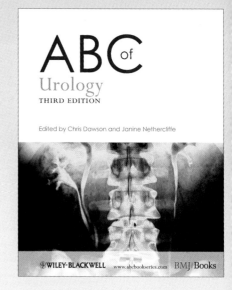

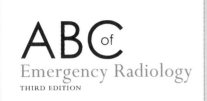
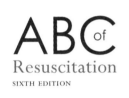
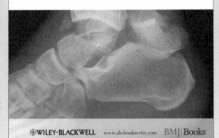
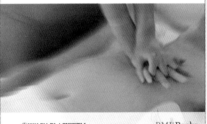

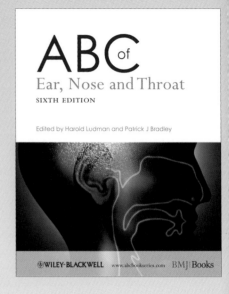
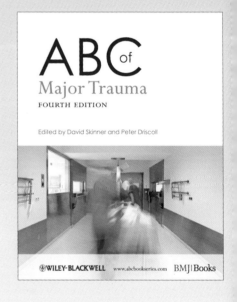

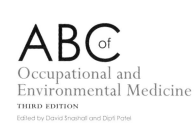

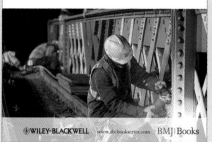

ABC of Occupational and Environmental Medicine

3RD EDITION

David Snashall & Dipti Patel
Guy's & St. Thomas' Hospital, London; Medical Advisory Service for Travellers Abroad (MASTA)

Since the publication of last edition, there have been huge changes in the world of occupational health. It has become firmly a part of international public health, and in Britain there is now a National Director for Work and Health. This fully updated new edition embraces these changes and:

- Provides comprehensive guidance on current occupational and environmental health practice and legislation
- Concentrates on the newer kinds of occupational disease, for example 'RSI', pesticide poisoning and electromagnetic radiation, where exposure and effects are difficult to understand
- Places an emphasis on work, health and well-being, and the public health benefits of work, the value of work, disabled people at work, the aging workforce, and vocational rehabilitation
- Includes chapters on the health effects of climate change and of occupational health and safety in relation to migration and terrorism

NOVEMBER 2012 | 9781444338171 | 168 PAGES | £27.99/US$44.95/€38.90/AU$52.95

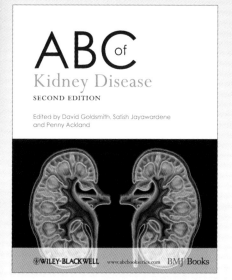

ABC of Kidney Disease

2ND EDITION

David Goldsmith, Satish Jayawardene & Penny Ackland
Guy's & St. Thomas' Hospital, London; King's College Hospital, London; Melbourne Grove Medical Practice, London

Nephrology is sometimes considered a complicated and specialized topic and the illustrative ABC format will help GPs quickly and easily assimilate the information needed. *ABC of Kidney Disease, 2nd Edition*:

- Is a practical guide to the most common renal diseases to enable non-renal health care workers to screen, identify, treat and refer renal patients appropriately and to provide the best possible care
- Covers organizational aspects of renal disease management, dialysis and transplantation
- Provides an explanatory glossary of renal terms, guidance on anaemia management and information on drug prescribing and interactions
- Has been fully revised in accordance with new guidelines

OCTOBER 2012 | 9780470672044 | 112 PAGES | £27.99/US$44.95/€35.90/AU$52.95

ALSO AVAILABLE

ABC of Adolescence
Russell Viner
2005 | 9780727915740 | 56 PAGES
£26.99 / US$41.95 / €34.90 / AU$52.95

ABC of Antithrombotic Therapy
Gregory Y. H. Lip & Andrew D. Blann
2003 | 9780727917713 | 67 PAGES
£26.50 / US$41.95 / €34.90 / AU$52.95

ABC of Arterial and Venous Disease, 2nd Edition
Richard Donnelly & Nick J. M. London
2009 | 9781405178891 | 120 PAGES
£31.50 / US$54.95 / €40.90 / AU$59.95

ABC of Asthma, 6th Edition
John Rees, Dipak Kanabar & Shriti Pattani
2009 | 9781405185967 | 104 PAGES
£26.99 / US$41.95 / €34.90 / AU$52.95

ABC of Burns
Shehan Hettiaratchy, Remo Papini & Peter Dziewulski
2004 | 9780727917874 | 56 PAGES
£26.50 / US$41.95 / €34.90 / AU$52.95

ABC of Child Protection, 4th Edition
Roy Meadow, Jacqueline Mok & Donna Rosenberg
2007 | 9780727918178 | 120 PAGES
£35.50 / US$59.95 / €45.90 / AU$67.95

ABC of Clinical Electrocardiography, 2nd Edition
Francis Morris, William J. Brady & John Camm
2008 | 9781405170642 | 112 PAGES
£34.50 / US$57.95 / €44.90 / AU$67.95

ABC of Clinical Genetics, 3rd Edition
Helen M. Kingston
2002 | 9780727916273 | 120 PAGES
£34.50 / US$57.95 / €44.90 / AU$67.95

ABC of Clinical Haematology, 3rd Edition
Drew Provan
2007 | 9781405153539 | 112 PAGES
£34.50 / US$59.95 / €44.90 / AU$67.95

ABC of Clinical Leadership
Tim Swanwick & Judy McKimm
2010 | 9781405198172 | 88 PAGES
£20.95 / US$32.95 / €26.90 / AU$39.95

ABC of Complementary Medicine, 2nd Edition
Catherine Zollman, Andrew J. Vickers & Janet Richardson
2008 | 9781405136570 | 64 PAGES
£28.95 / US$47.95 / €37.90 / AU$54.95

ABC of COPD, 2nd Edition
Graeme P. Currie
2010 | 9781444333886 | 88 PAGES
£23.95 / US$37.95 / €30.90 / AU$47.95

ABC of Dermatology, 5th Edition
Paul K. Buxton & Rachael Morris-Jones
2009 | 9781405170659 | 224 PAGES
£34.50 / US$58.95 / €44.90 / AU$67.95

ABC of Diabetes, 6th Edition
Tim Holt & Sudhesh Kumar
2007 | 9781405177849 | 112 PAGES
£31.50 / US$52.95 / €40.90 / AU$59.95

ABC of Eating Disorders
Jane Morris
2008 | 9780727918437 | 80 PAGES
£26.50 / US$41.95 / €34.90 / AU$52.95

ABC of Emergency Differential Diagnosis
Francis Morris & Alan Fletcher
2009 | 9781405170635 | 96 PAGES
£31.50 / US$55.95 / €40.90 / AU$59.95

ABC of Geriatric Medicine
Nicola Cooper, Kirsty Forrest & Graham Mulley
2009 | 9781405169424 | 88 PAGES
£26.50 / US$44.95 / €34.90 / AU$52.95

ABC of Headache
Anne MacGregor & Alison Frith
2008 | 9781405170666 | 88 PAGES
£23.95 / US$41.95 / €30.90 / AU$47.95

ABC of Heart Failure, 2nd Edition
Russell C. Davis, Michael K. Davis & Gregory Y. H. Lip
2006 | 9780727916440 | 72 PAGES
£26.50 / US$41.95 / €34.90 / AU$52.95

ABC of Imaging in Trauma
Leonard J. King & David C. Wherry
2008 | 9781405183321 | 144 PAGES
£31.50 / US$50.95 / €40.90 / AU$59.95

ABC of Interventional Cardiology, 2nd Edition
Ever D. Grech
2010 | 9781405170673 | 120 PAGES
£25.95 / US$40.95 / €33.90 / AU$49.95

ABC of Learning and Teaching in Medicine, 2nd Edition
Peter Cantillon & Diana Wood
2009 | 9781405185974 | 96 PAGES
£22.99 / US$35.95 / €29.90 / AU$44.95

ABC of Liver, Pancreas and Gall Bladder
Ian Beckingham
1905 | 9780727915313 | 64 PAGES
£24.95 / US$39.95 / €32.90 / AU$47.95

ABC of Lung Cancer
Ian Hunt, Martin M. Muers & Tom Treasure
2009 | 9781405146524 | 64 PAGES
£25.95 / US$41.95 / €33.90 / AU$49.95

ABC of Medical Law
Lorraine Corfield, Ingrid Granne & William Latimer-Sayer
2009 | 9781405176286 | 64 PAGES
£24.95 / US$39.95 / €32.90 / AU$47.95

ABC of Mental Health, 2nd Edition
Teifion Davies & Tom Craig
2009 | 9780727916396 | 128 PAGES
£32.50 / US$52.95 / €41.90 / AU$62.95

ABC of Obesity
Naveed Sattar & Mike Lean
2007 | 9781405136747 | 64 PAGES
£24.99 / US$39.99 / €32.90 / AU$47.95

ABC of One to Seven, 5th Edition
Bernard Valman
2009 | 9781405181051 | 168 PAGES
£32.50 / US$52.95 / €41.90 / AU$62.95

ABC of Palliative Care, 2nd Edition
Marie Fallon & Geoffrey Hanks
2006 | 9781405130790 | 96 PAGES
£30.50 / US$52.95 / €39.90 / AU$57.95

ABC of Patient Safety
John Sandars & Gary Cook
2007 | 9781405156929 | 64 PAGES
£28.50 / US$46.99 / €36.90 / AU$54.95

ABC of Practical Procedures
Tim Nutbeam & Ron Daniels
2009 | 9781405185950 | 144 PAGES
£31.50 / US$50.95 / €40.90 / AU$59.95

ABC of Preterm Birth
William McGuire & Peter Fowlie
2005 | 9780727917638 | 56 PAGES
£26.50 / US$41.95 / €34.90 / AU$52.95

ABC of Psychological Medicine
Richard Mayou, Michael Sharpe & Alan Carson
2003 | 9780727915566 | 72 PAGES
£26.99 / US$41.95 / €34.90 / AU$52.95

ABC of Rheumatology, 4th Edition
Ade Adebajo
2009 | 9781405170680 | 192 PAGES
£31.95 / US$50.95 / €41.90 / AU$62.95

ABC of Sepsis
Ron Daniels & Tim Nutbeam
2009 | 9781405181945 | 104 PAGES
£31.50 / US$52.95 / €40.90 / AU$59.95

ABC of Sexual Health, 2nd Edition
John Tomlinson
2004 | 9780727917591 | 96 PAGES
£31.50 / US$52.95 / €40.90 / AU$59.95

ABC of Skin Cancer
Sajjad Rajpar & Jerry Marsden
2008 | 9781405162197 | 80 PAGES
£26.50 / US$47.95 / €34.90 / AU$52.95

ABC of Spinal Disorders
Andrew Clarke, Alwyn Jones & Michael O'Malley
2009 | 9781405170697 | 72 PAGES
£24.95 / US$39.95 / €32.90 / AU$47.95

ABC of Sports and Exercise Medicine, 3rd Edition
Gregory Whyte, Mark Harries & Clyde Williams
2005 | 9780727918130 | 136 PAGES
£34.95 / US$62.95 / €44.90 / AU$67.95

ABC of Subfertility
Peter Braude & Alison Taylor
2005 | 9780727915344 | 64 PAGES
£24.95 / US$39.95 / €32.90 / AU$47.95

ABC of the First Year, 6th Edition
Bernard Valman & Roslyn Thomas
2009 | 9781405180375 | 136 PAGES
£31.50 / US$55.95 / €40.90 / AU$59.95

ABC of the Upper Gastrointestinal Tract
Robert Logan, Adam Harris & J. J. Misiewicz
2002 | 9780727912664 | 54 PAGES
£26.50 / US$41.95 / €34.90 / AU$52.95

ABC of Transfusion, 4th Edition
Marcela Contreras
2009 | 9781405156462 | 128 PAGES
£31.50 / US$55.95 / €40.90 / AU$59.95

ABC of Tubes, Drains, Lines and Frames
Adam Brooks, Peter F. Mahoney & Brian Rowlands
2008 | 9781405160148 | 88 PAGES
£26.50 / US$41.95 / €34.90 / AU$52.95

For more information on any of our medical books, please visit **www.wiley.com/go/medicine**